PORCINE ENZOOTIC PNEUMONIA

Beatriz García-Morante, Joaquim Segalés
and Marina Sibila

SERVET

Plaza Antonio Beltrán Martínez nº 1, planta 8 - letra I
(Centro empresarial El Trovador)
50002 Zaragoza - Spain

First printing: November 2018

This book has been published originally in Spanish under the title:
Neumonía enzoótica porcina
© 2018 Grupo Asís Biomedia, S.L.
ISBN Spanish edition: 978-84-17225-00-1

Translation:
Chef du Monde S.L., Barcelona (Spain)
Illustrator:
Jacob Gragera Artal

ISBN: 978-84-17225-57-5
D.L.: Z 515-2018

Design, layout and printing:
Servet editorial - Grupo Asís Biomedia, S.L.
www.grupoasis.com
nfo@grupoasis.com

Servet is the publishing house of Grupo Asís

Warning:
Veterinary science is constantly evolving, as are pharmacology and the other sciences. Inevitably, it is therefore the responsibility of the veterinary surgeon to determine and verify the dosage, the method of administration, the duration of treatment and any possible contraindications to the treatments given to each individual patient, based on his or her professional experience. Neither the publisher nor the author can be held liable for any damage or harm caused to people, animals or properties resulting from the correct or incorrect application of the information contained in this book.

THE AUTHORS

Beatriz García-Morante

Beatriz García-Morante graduated from the Autonomous University of Barcelona (UAB) with a degree in veterinary medicine in 2012, and gained an interuniversity Master's Degree in Advanced Immunology from the UAB and the University of Barcelona (UB) in 2013. She earned her PhD under the Government of Catalonia's Industrial Doctorates Plan in 2017, in a collaborative arrangement between the pharmaceutical industry and CReSA (Centre de Recerca en Sanitat Animal; Centre for Animal Health Research) at IRTA (Institut de Recerca i Tecnologia Agroalimentaries; Institute of Agri-Food Research and Technology), located on the UAB campus. Her doctoral thesis sought improvements to the experimental model for the study of *Mycoplasma hyopneumoniae* infection, under the supervision of Dr Marina Sibila and Dr Joaquim Segalés. She has published articles in national and international journals, and has also been a resident of the European College of Porcine Health and Management (ECPHM) since 2015, mentored by Dr Sergio López and Dr Joaquim Segalés.

Joaquim Segalés

Joaquim Segalés graduated in veterinary medicine from the UAB in 1991 and was awarded his PhD by the same university in 1996, after spending 15 months at the University of Minnesota (UM) in the USA, codirected by Dr Mariano Domingo (UAB) and Dr Carlos Pijoan (UM). He became a diplomate of the European College of Veterinary Pathologists (ECVP) in 2000 and by the ECPHM in 2004. He is a founding member of the ECPHM and was its president between 2013 and 2016. Dr Segalés is a tenured lecturer at the Department of Animal Health and Anatomy of the Faculty of Veterinary Medicine at the UAB, and he is also a researcher with CReSA–IRTA, where he was director between 2012 and 2017.

He participates in many Spanish and European research projects, and collaborates with Spanish and international companies in the pig production sector. His research includes porcine respiratory and reproductive syndrome virus (PRRSV), *Haemophilus parasuis*, Aujeszky's disease virus (ADV), *Mycoplasma hyopneumoniae*, hepatitis E virus, torque teno sus virus (TTSuV), and diseases associated with porcine circovirus type 2 (PCV2). He is coauthor of over 270 articles in international scientific journals, 10 chapters of internationally acclaimed books, a book on pig necropsy, and 3 books on clinical cases in pigs.

Marina Sibila

Marina Sibila graduated in biological sciences from the UB in 1999. Under the supervision of Dr Maria Calsamiglia, she completed her PhD on the molecular epidemiology of *M. hyopneumoniae* infection at the Faculty of Veterinary Medicine of the UAB in 2004. She is currently a researcher at CReSA-IRTA, where she is continuing her work on *M. hyopneumoniae* and other pig pathogens, including PCV2, PRRSV, *Haemophilus parasuis, Actinobacillus pleuropneumoniae, Mycoplasma hyorhinis*, and TTSuV. Her research includes molecular epidemiology, the development of experimental models and diagnostic tools, and vaccine efficacy studies. Dr Sibila collaborates in many Spanish and international research projects, and she has published more than 60 scientific and educational articles. She is also co-author of a book chapter on the evaluation of lung lesions in pigs at the abattoir and a handbook of laboratory diagnosis in pigs. Dr Sibila has participated as a speaker at various conferences in the sector, both in Spain and internationally, and her teaching activities have included PhD courses and classes for a master's degree in swine health and production and directing various doctoral theses.

CONTENTS

1

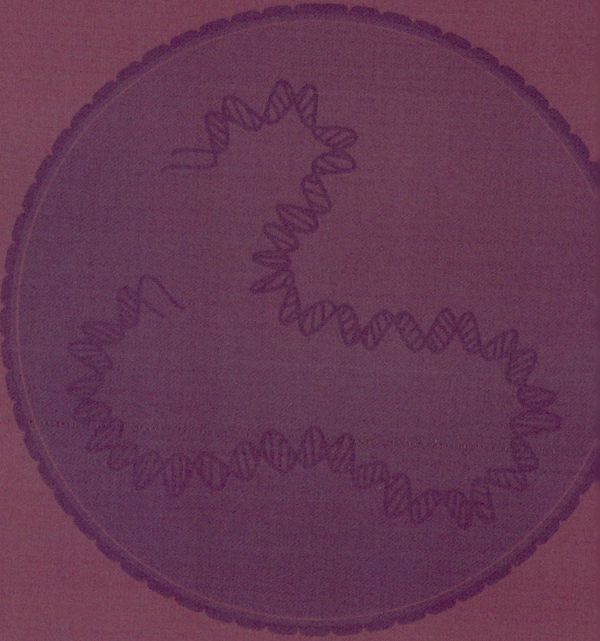

MYCOPLASMA HYOPNEUMONIAE, PRIMARY AGENT

SOME HISTORY...

Although chronic pneumonia was first recognised in pigs more than a century ago, it was not until the 1930s when progress started towards a better understanding of its aetiology. In fact, what are now known as porcine mycoplasmosis (PM) and swine influenza were not clearly separated and recognised as separate disease entities until the 1950s. It was initially thought that PM was caused by a virus, so it was called "viral pneumonia".

PM was reproduced experimentally for the first time in 1965, almost simultaneously by Maré and Switzer in the United States, and Goodwin et al. in the United Kingdom. The isolate used by Maré and Switzer to reproduce the disease was called strain 11 (*Mycoplasma hyopneumoniae*), and the strain isolated by Goodwin was called strain J (*Mycoplasma suipneumoniae*). The name *M. hyopneumoniae* was chosen as the accepted species name, as it was the first name to be used, but strain J has been established as the *M. hyopneumoniae* type strain. Today, both strain 11 and strain J are considered to be reference strains and their main characteristics are summarised in Table 1.

Table 1. Current characteristics of *M. hyopneumoniae* reference strains.

	Strain J	Strain 11
Discovered by	Goodwin et al.	Maré and Switzer
Origin	United Kingdom	United States
Original culture	ATCC and NCTC	ATCC
Type strain	Yes	No
Pathogenicity	Nonpathogenic	Pathogenic[1]

ATCC: American Type Culture Collection; NCTC: National Collection of Type Cultures.

[1]Few studies have recently used strain 11 for experimental inoculation.

Some of the *M. hyopneumoniae* vaccines currently available on the market are based on the reference strains.

CHARACTERISTICS OF MYCOPLASMAS

Mycoplasma hyopneumoniae:

Kingdom: *Bacteria*

Phylum or division: *Firmicutes*

Class: *Mollicutes*

Order: *Mycoplasmatales*

Family: *Mycoplasmataceae*

Genus: *Mycoplasma*

The genus *Mycoplasma* is the subgroup with the greatest number of recognised species in the class *Mollicutes*. Mycoplasmas possess a series of characteristics that makes them unique amongst bacteria:

- They have no cell wall, and their outermost structure is a triple-layered cell membrane containing sterols.
- They are thought to be the smallest known organisms that are free-living and capable of self-replication.
- Their genome is small, with fewer genes than other bacteria and this reduces their metabolic and enzymatic capacity, which explains their pronounced nutritional needs, leading to their dependency on a host.

Mycoplasmas need sterols to maintain cell membrane stability and obtain them (including cholesterol) from the environment, usually from the animals that they infect.

Figure 1 shows the main characteristics of mycoplasmas, and Table 2 links these characteristics with their effects.

Figure 1. Diagram of the structure of *M. hyopneumoniae*. The particle is small (0.2–0.8 μm in diameter).
1: Small genome entails a significant reduction in the ability to biosynthesise.
2: No cell wall, but cell membrane containing sterols.

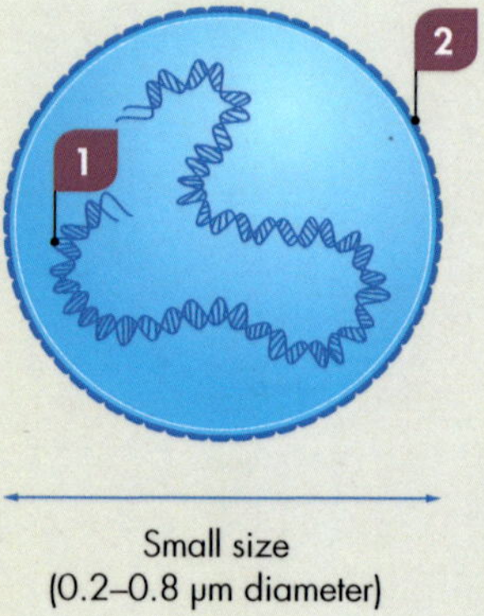

Other mycoplasmas are also commonly found in the pig respiratory tract, not only *M. hyopneumoniae*: *Mycoplasma hyorhinis*, which can also be involved in pneumonia, polyserositis and arthritis, and *Mycoplasma flocculare*, which is not associated with any disease. Other nonrespiratory mycoplasmas, such as *Mycoplasma hyosynoviae* and *Mycoplasma suis*, are also known to be pathogenic in pigs.

Table 2. Characteristics of mycoplasmas and their effects.

Characteristic	Effect
Lack cell wall	Not susceptible to antibiotics that act on the cell wall, such as the β-lactams (penicillins, cephalosporins, etc.).
	Do not stain with Gram stain.
	Pleomorphic, with ability to alter shape and size.
	Sensitive to environmental conditions. Mycoplasmas survive for a relatively short period outside the host.
Cell membrane contains sterols	Need to acquire sterols, such as cholesterol, either from the environment or the host, to grow.
Small size (≈0.2–0.8 μm diameter)	Colonies are invisible to the naked eye, requiring the use of a light microscope.
	Pass through filters that retain other bacteria.
Small genome	Drastically reduced ability to biosynthesise, hence their dependence on a suitable host or environment.

CULTURE AND ISOLATION

M. hyopneumoniae is one of the most difficult mycoplasmas to isolate and cultivate. The liquid medium most commonly used for this purpose was developed by Niels Friis in 1975. There are currently some variations on this medium in use, but these still contain one of the essential nutrients to encourage *M. hyopneumoniae* growth: cholesterol, which is sourced from animal serum, typically from pigs and/or horses. *M. hyopneumoniae* is usually isolated by resuspending part of the lung adjacent to an area affected by pneumonia in a suitable liquid medium. It is common practice to perform various blind subcultures in a liquid medium before inoculating a solid medium, as *M. hyopneumoniae* does not usually grow on solid mediums on primary isolation. The enriched medium required to culture *M. hyopneumoniae* is also easily contaminated by other bacteria that inhabit the pig's respiratory tract, especially *M. hyorhinis*, and also by commensal organisms.

Growth of *M. hyopneumoniae* in the liquid culture medium produces turbidity and acidifies the medium, so phenol red (a pH indicator) is often added to make pathogen growth visible, by a gradual change in the colour of the medium, from an original dark red to a yellowish–orange colour. This characteristic allows the *M. hyopneumoniae* culture to be titrated, and the result is expressed in colour changing units, or CCU (Figs. 2 and 3).

Figure 2. Diagram of *M. hyopneumoniae* culture titration by endpoint dilution assay, expressed as CCU/ml.

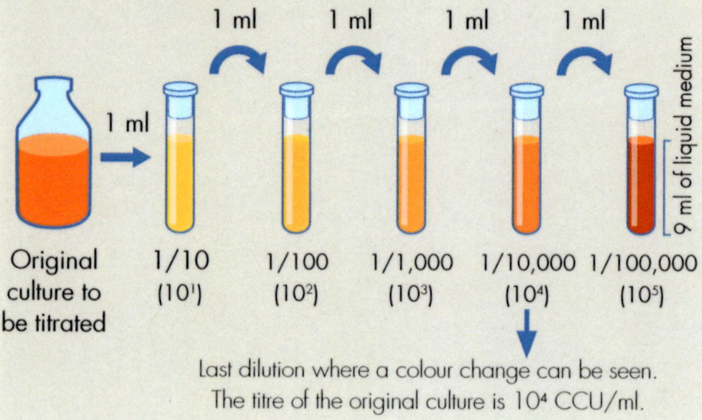

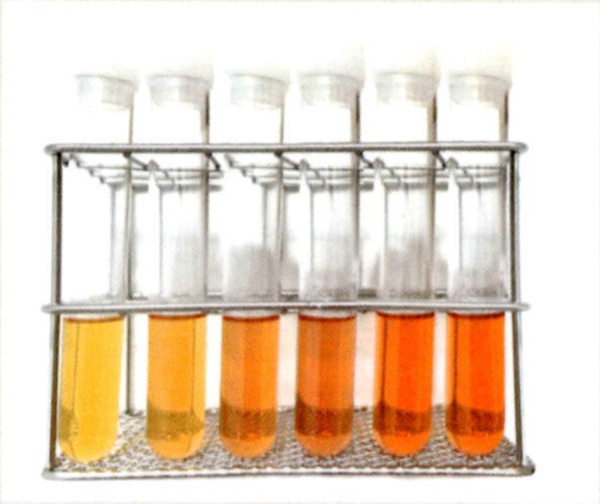

Figure 3. Titration of *M. hyopneumoniae* culture by endpoint dilution assay.

In a solid medium, *M. hyopneumoniae* colonies tend to lack the classic fried-egg shape of other *Mollicutes* colonies, as they do not usually have a defined centre and tend to look granular (Fig. 4); their structure may sometimes be irregular and asymmetrical.

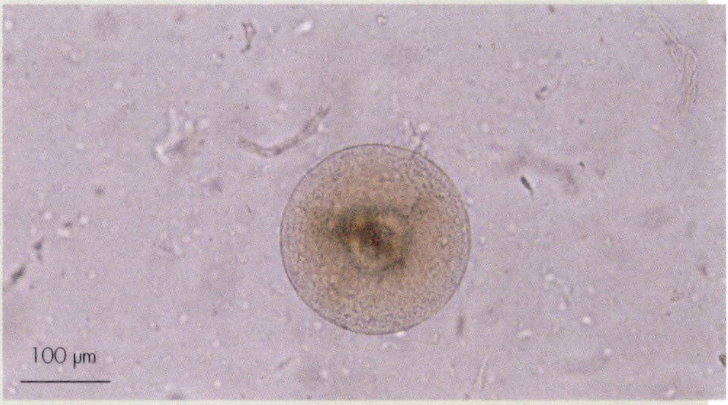

Figure 4. *M. hyopneumoniae* colony observed at 100× with a light microscope.

> *M. hyopneumoniae* is considered to be a facultative anaerobe micro-organism. Tubes of liquid medium are incubated at 37 °C under aerobic conditions; plates of solid medium are also incubated at 37 °C, but in microaerobiosis with 5 % carbon dioxide (CO_2).

PATHOGENESIS OF *M. HYOPNEUMONIAE* INFECTION

M. hyopneumoniae is an important pathogenic micro-organism in pigs. Colonization of the pig's respiratory tract is essential to start the infection. *M. hyopneumoniae* enters the airways and mainly adheres to the cilia of the epithelial cells, causing ciliostasis (loss of motility), deciliation (loss of cilia) and resulting death of the affected ciliated epithelial cells and the goblet cells (which produce mucus) (Fig. 5). This impairment of the mucociliary system causes major disruption of the respiratory tract's defen-

> Adhesins are proteins anchored to the *M. hyopneumoniae* outer membrane, which facilitate adhesion of the bacteria to the cilia of the epithelial cells in the pig's respiratory tract. These cilia contain receptors to this pathogen.

sive capabilities, which are extremely important to control concomitant pathogens.

One important characteristic of *M. hyopneumoniae* infection is the inflammatory response that is generated. As the infection advances and spreads, macrophages and lymphocytes migrate and infiltrate the affected airways, producing various cytokines that promote mobilisation of more immune system cells. These inflammatory cells restrict the flow of air and tend to be unable to eliminate the pathogen quickly or effectively, leading to chronic colonisation of the airways and a prolonged local inflammatory response that is closely linked to the development of lung lesions.

> In the case of *M. hyopneumoniae*, immunopathological events are decisive in the development of lung lesions, but the exact mechanisms causing these processes are still unknown.

> Tissue damage caused by inflammation, decreased diameter of the lower respiratory airways and an altered immune response are major contributors to the characteristic chronic nature of *M. hyopneumoniae* infection.

Figure 5. Simplified diagram of (a) normal respiratory epithelium in a pig and (b) how this is affected by *M. hyopneumoniae* infection.

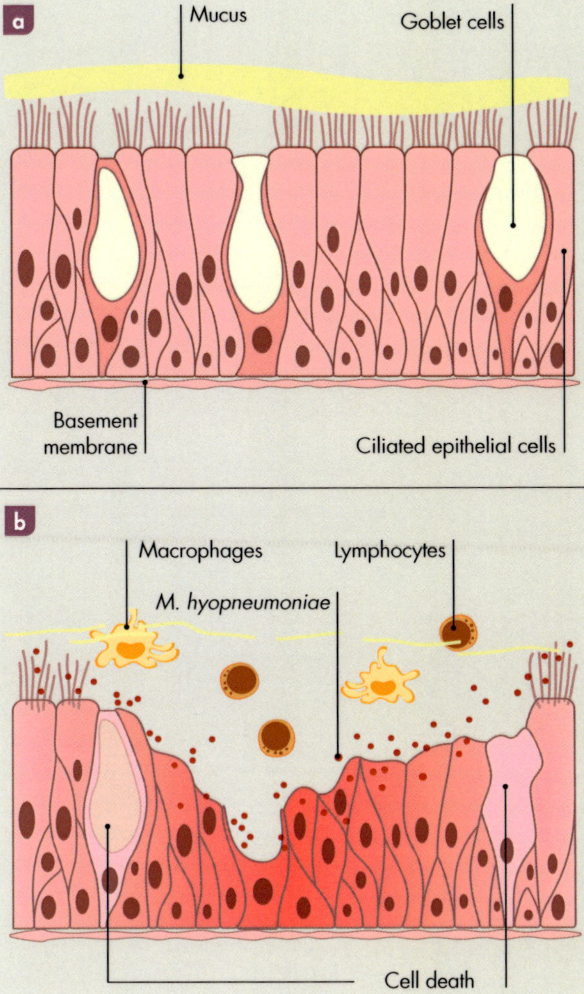

DISEASES ASSOCIATED WITH *M. HYOPNEUMONIAE* INFECTION

M. hyopneumoniae is a respiratory pathogen that can only infect domestic pigs (*Sus scrofa domesticus*) and wild boar (*Sus scrofa*). It is considered to be a primary pathogen, as it can cause disease by itself, but it usually interacts with other pathogenic agents to cause respiratory disease in pigs (Fig. 6). *M. hyopneumoniae* can be involved in three distinct disease entities:

- **Porcine mycoplasmosis (PM):** infection by *M. hyopneumoniae* alone. This is very rare and is practically restricted to experimental conditions or immunologically naive herds.
- **Enzootic pneumonia (EP):** coinfection with *M. hyopneumoniae* as the primary pathogen and other bacteria as concomitant pathogen(s).
- **Porcine respiratory disease complex (PRDC):** coinfection with various viral and bacterial pig pathogens, often including *M. hyopneumoniae*.

> EP is caused by bacterial coinfection, with *M. hyopneumoniae* as the primary agent, but PRDC involves coinfection by multiple pathogens, where *M. hyopneumoniae* may or may not be present.

Figure 6. Outline of the pig pathogens most frequently involved in EP and PRDC in the cases of coinfection with *M. hyopneumoniae*.

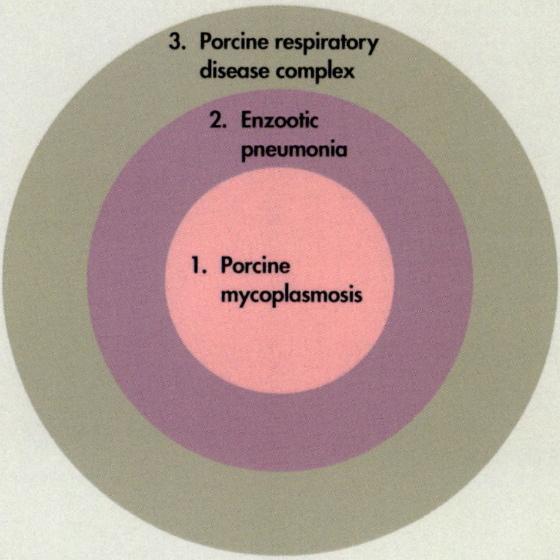

1. Porcine mycoplasmosis
   - *Mycoplasma hyopneumoniae*

2. Enzootic pneumonia
   - *Bordetella bronchiseptica*
   - *Streptococcus suis*
   - *Trueperella pyogenes*
   - *Pasteurella multocida*
   - *Actinobacillus pleuropneumoniae*
   - *Mycoplasma hyorhinis*
   - *Haemophilus parasuis*

3. Porcine respiratory disease complex
   - Porcine reproductive and respiratory syndrome virus
   - Swine influenza virus
   - Porcine circovirus type 2
   - Aujeszky's disease virus
   - Porcine respiratory coronavirus

2

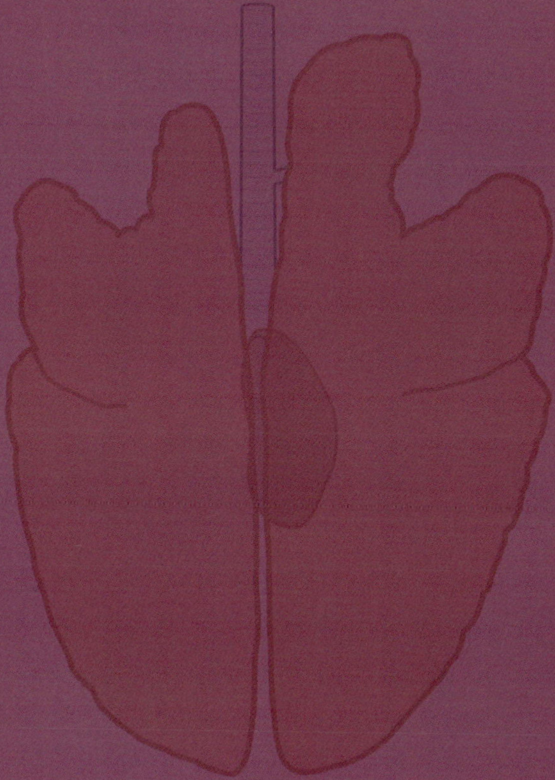

WHAT ARE THE CLINICAL SIGNS OF *M. HYOPNEUMONIAE* INFECTION?

CLINICAL DIAGNOSIS

Coughing and dyspnoea are the main clinical signs of respiratory diseases. They can be caused by a wide variety of infectious agents, and modified by coinfections and environmental factors. Their aetiology is quite unspecific. A dry, nonproductive cough in fattening pigs is a clinical sign that is consistent with the diseases associated with *M. hyopneumoniae*.

A nonproductive dry cough is suggestive of, but not exclusive to, *M. hyopneumoniae* infection.

Under experimental conditions, coughing tends to start 2 weeks postinfection (p.i.), although this incubation period can vary from 1 to 3 weeks. However, this period can vary considerably in the field, and can be as long as 6 weeks. Coughing can last between 1 week and 2 months under both experimental and farm conditions. It is important to remember that subclinical *M. hyopneumoniae* infections are common and are not linked to any obvious clinical signs.

A noncomplicated *M. hyopneumoniae* infection causes a nonproductive dry cough of chronic nature and mainly affects fatteners. The disease is characterised by high morbidity, low mortality and has a limited effect on the animal's productive performance.

M. hyopneumoniae infection encourages coinfection by other respiratory pathogens, leading to enzootic pneumonia (EP) or porcine respiratory disease complex (PRDC), so the respiratory disease often worsens. In these cases, dyspnoea and fever can be seen in addition to coughing; morbidity and mortality can increase, affecting the animal's productive performance significantly. Two forms of EP can be distinguished, according to the clinical expression of the disease: the endemic form and the epidemic form (Table 1).

Table 1. Summary of the clinical characteristics of endemic and epidemic EP.

	Endemic EP	Epidemic EP
Incidence	High	Low
Type	Chronic	Acute
Morbidity	High	Very high
Mortality	Very low	Medium–low
Where?	Herds that are immunologically positive for *M. hyopneumoniae*, whether through vaccination or continual field exposure.	Herds that are immunologically negative for *M. hyopneumoniae*. Introduction of *M. hyopneumoniae* into farms previously free of the disease and unvaccinated.
Who?	Animals over 6 weeks of age, especially during the fattening stage.	Animals of all ages, but usually during fattening.
Clinical signs	Subclinical presentation, or nonproductive dry cough with a gradual onset. Other more severe signs tend to be the result of concomitant infections.	Nonproductive dry cough with sudden onset. Other more severe signs tend to be the result of concomitant infections.
Productive performance	Production parameters are not always affected. If they do change, slow growth rate, poor feed conversion rate, uneven growth in the litter or pen, and a protracted late fattening phase can be seen.	Production parameters tend to be affected because there is often a loss of appetite in the affected pens. The parameters affected are the same as in the endemic form, although more severe.

The clinical expression of EP will largely depend on the immune status of the animal infected by *M. hyopneumoniae*. If the animal has been infected before and/or has been vaccinated, it will probably show signs of the endemic form. Conversely, animals with no immunity will probably exhibit the epidemic form. In Europe, especially in the densely populated pig producing areas, the endemic form is the most common, due to continuous circulation of *M. hyopneumoniae* between farms and widespread vaccination.

Not all *M. hyopneumoniae* infections result in EP. In fact, one of the most important aspects of *M. hyopneumoniae* infection is its ability to cause subclinical, chronic and often persistent infection.

PATHOLOGICAL DIAGNOSIS

Lung lesions consistent with *M. hyopneumoniae* infection can have other causes, so an exhaustive assessment of these lesions must be made.

Although the macroscopic and microscopic lesions are highly consistent with *M. hyopneumoniae* infection, these are not exclusive, as various infectious agents and some non-biological factors can also cause or facilitate them.

MACROSCOPIC LUNG LESIONS

Porcine mycoplasmosis (PM) is characterised by areas of pulmonary consolidation, often well demarcated and more collapsed than the surrounding lung tissue of healthy appearance. It mainly affects the areas of the lung (apical and cardiac lobes, and the cranial portions of the diaphragmatic lobes). Lesions also tend to be seen in the accessory lobe. The affected area can be distinguished visually as it acquires a dark red to greyish red colour, according to the chronology of the lesion. This macroscopic pattern is called cranioventral pulmonary consolidation (CVPC) (Fig. 1).

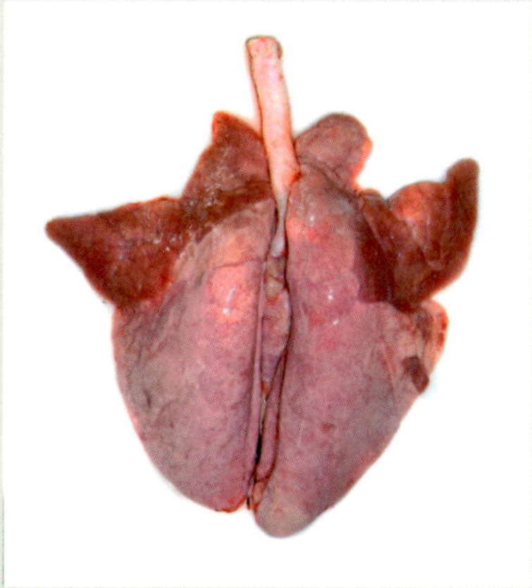

Figure 1. Dorsal view of a pig lung showing lesions consistent with *M. hyopneumoniae* infection. CVPC can been seen, affecting the left apical lobe, and both cardiac lobes. The right diaphragmatic lobe appears mildly affected.

Experimentally, CVPC has been seen from the first week p.i. onwards, reaching its maximum spread and severity approximately 4 weeks p.i. However, these lesions tend to resolve about 8 weeks p.i., sometimes forming fissures of fibrous tissue with shrinkage of lung tissue.

In PM, when the surface of an area of consolidated lung tissue is sectioned, a catarrhal exudate can be seen in the airways. Conversely, when a mucopurulent exudate can be seen, the involvement of other respiratory pathogens is guaranteed, and the animal is probably suffering from EP. It is important to remember that *M. hyopneumoniae* infection is not the only cause of CVPC; other organisms, especially *Pasteurella multocida* and swine influenza virus, can also give rise to very similar lung lesions.

Assessment of CVPC usually involves the determination of its extent, and various methods can provide a value for the severity of the lesions. The most widely used systems for quantifying CVPC, and their main characteristics, are shown in Table 2.

Table 2. Methods of CVPC quantification described in the scientific literature. Adapted from García-Morante et al., (2016).

Reference	Description	Maximum score	Visual representation (max. score/lobe)
Goodwin et al. (1969)	Quantification of the affected area from 0–10, or 0–5, depending on the lobe. Lobe scores are added to give a total score for the area of lung affected.	55 points	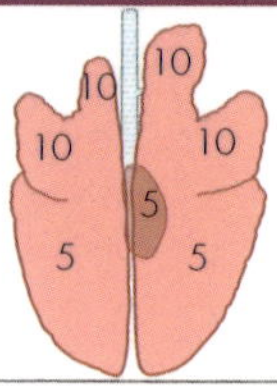
Hannan et al. (1982)	Affected area represented on a lung diagram. The number of triangles affected per lobe are multiplied by 5 and divided by the total number of triangles in each lobe. Lobe scores are added to give a total score for the area of lung affected.	35 points **1.** 4	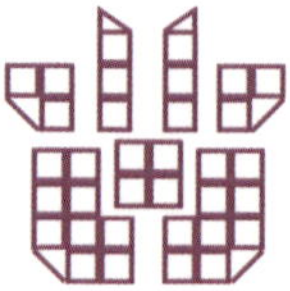
Madec and Kobisch (1982)	Quantification of the affected area using four categories: 0. No lesion. 1. Lesions affecting <25 % of the lobe surface. 2. Lesions affecting 25–49 % of the lobe surface. 3. Lesions affecting 50–74 % of the lobe surface. 4. Lesions affecting ≥75 % of the lobe surface. Lobe scores are added to give a total score for the area of lung affected.	28 points	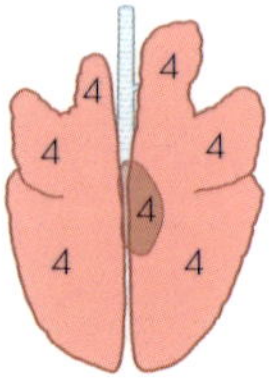

▶

Reference	Description	Maximum score	Visual representation (max. score/lobe)
Straw et al. (1986)	The percentage of the area of each lobe affected is multiplied by the relative size of the lobe and added together to give the percentage of the total area of lung affected.	100 %	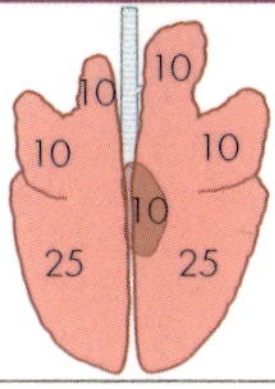
Image analysis	Quantification of the area of lung affected from an image of the lung (photo). The area of the lesion and the total lung area are delineated in the image and analysed digitally to determine the proportion of the lung area affected.	100 %	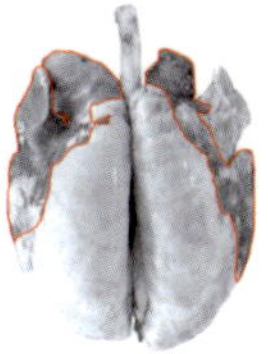
Morrison et al. (1985)	The percentage of the area of each lobe affected is multiplied by the relative weight of the lobe and added together to give the percentage of the total weight of lung affected.	100 %	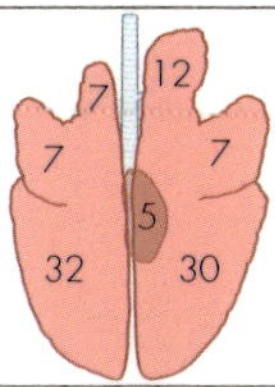
Christensen et al. (1999)	The percentage of the area of each lobe affected is multiplied by the relative weight of the lobe and added together to give the percentage of the total weight of lung affected. Separate scores are given to the cranial area of the diaphragmatic lobes.	100 %	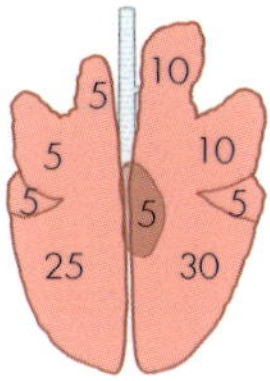
Ph. Eur.[1](2013)	The percentage of the area of each lobe affected is multiplied by the relative weight of the lobe and added together to give the percentage of the total weight of lung affected.	100 %	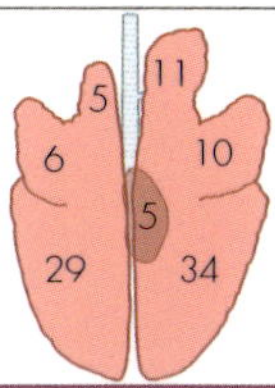

[1]*European Pharmacopoeia.*

Lung inspection at the abattoir is useful to detect lesions consistent with *M. hyopneumoniae* infection. Small lesions can be associated with subclinical respiratory infections that tend to have an adverse effect on production in pigs. However, it is difficult to reach a diagnosis based only on examination of the lungs at the abattoir as these lesions lack specificity and may become chronic over time.

MICROSCOPIC LUNG LESIONS

Microscopic lesions mainly consist of bronchointerstitial pneumonia (BIP), with significant cellular infiltration (mainly lymphocytes and macrophages) at the peribronchial and perivascular levels, and in the bronchoalveolar spaces (Fig. 2). As the infection progresses, hyperplasia (follicle formation) of the bronchus-associated lymphoid tissue (BALT) can be seen. When other respiratory pathogens are involved, this BIP develops rapidly to a suppurative or purulent bronchopneumonia, with a predominantly neutrophilic exudate in the alveoli and airways.

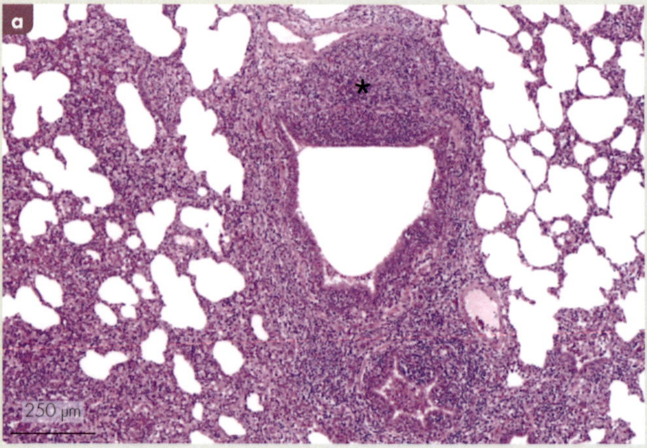

Lung lesions are probably a consequence of the host's immune response to the infection, and not caused by *M. hyopneumoniae* itself.

Dry and persistent coughing in fatteners of any stage and postmortem findings of CVPC, sometimes accompanied by reduced performance, lead to the following differential diagnosis:

- PM or EP.
- Swine influenza.
- Pneumonic pasteurellosis (this tends to be secondary to the two conditions listed above, or to other problems, such as porcine reproductive and respiratory syndrome [PRRS]).

The involvement of these pathogens in the clinical presentation and/or lesions should be confirmed by laboratory tests.

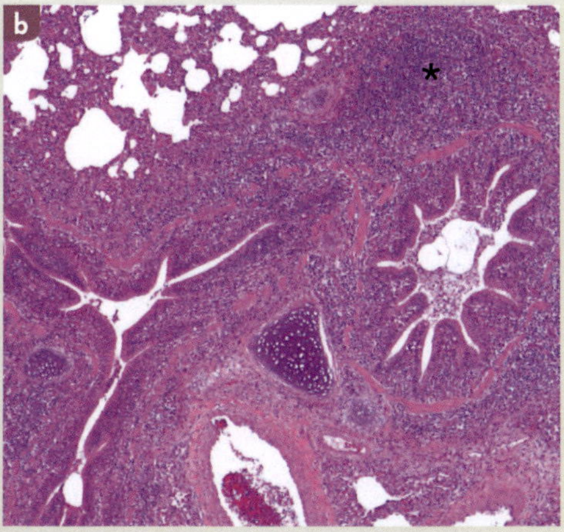

Figure 2. Microscopic images (a and b) of a pig lung showing lesions consistent with *M. hyopneumoniae* infection, showing BIP with formation of peribronchial and peribronchiolar lymphoid follicles (asterisk).

LABORATORY DIAGNOSIS

Many laboratory techniques can be used to detect and monitor *M. hyopneumoniae* infection, all of which focus on detecting the pathogen directly or indirectly (Table 3). These techniques are presented below, along with their advantages and principal limitations.

> The clinical signs and postmortem examination, combined with histopathological analysis, can provide a presumptive diagnosis of the agents involved. Diagnostic techniques that prove the presence of the pathogen, or past contact with it, are used for definitive confirmation of the disease.

All laboratory techniques have limitations, so it is advisable to combine several techniques in order to provide the best information, and optimise diagnostic precision.

DETECTING THE PATHOGEN

Isolation of the bacterium has been considered for many years to be the reference technique, or gold standard, to diagnose *M. hyopneumoniae*, as it is the only method that clearly demonstrates the involvement of the pathogen in lung lesions. However, it is currently not performed routinely due to:

- Low sensitivity. A negative result does not rule out infection.
- Requires specialised culture media.
- Slow growth (3 weeks or more to confirm the pathogen's presence).
- High rates of contamination with other bacteria, especially *M. hyorhinis*, which is a common coloniser of the pig's respiratory tract.

Table 3. Main characteristics of the laboratory techniques used to diagnose *M. hyopneumoniae* infection.

Technique	Detects	Sensitivity	Specificity	Substrate	Availability	Price	Time
Bacterial culture	Viable organism	red	green	Lung tissue or BALF[1]	red	red	red
IHC	Antigen	yellow	yellow	Lung tissue	red	yellow	yellow
IF	Antigen	yellow	yellow	Lung tissue	red	yellow	yellow
ISH	DNA	yellow	green	Lung tissue	red	yellow	yellow
PCR	DNA	green	green	Multiple substrates	green	yellow	green
ELISA	Antibodies	green	yellow	Blood (serum)	green	green	green

Bronchoalveolar lavage fluid. Legend: green: very good; yellow: good; red: moderate.

M. hyopneumoniae is therefore cultured and isolated under very specific circumstances, notably in research. It is also worth remembering that only a few specialised laboratories perform this technique.

M. hyopneumoniae culture is not recommended as a routine diagnostic technique. A negative result in the samples tested when trying to isolate the organism should not be used to rule out the presence or involvement of *M. hyopneumoniae*.

DETECTING THE ANTIGEN

Immunohistochemistry (IHC) and immunofluorescence (IF) are both based on the bond between *M. hyopneumoniae* antigens in the lung tissue and specific antibodies, which enables visualisation of *M. hyopneumoniae* if present in the lesions observed. Both techniques are performed on sections of lung tissue (fixed in formalin and embedded in paraffin, or frozen), although they differ in the ways that they visualise or detect the antigens. In IHC (Fig. 3) the antigen–antibody reaction is visualised through a colorimetric enzymatic reaction, and in IF the antibodies are labelled with a fluorescent substance. The use of immunological techniques for diagnosis is quite rare, as they have the following limitations:

- Can only be used postmortem.
- Low sensitivity.
- Complicated sample processing.
- Specificity can be affected by cross-reaction between the antibodies used and other mycoplasmas, such as *M. flocculare*.

As with bacterial isolation, few laboratories specialise in these techniques, so they do not tend to be used in routine diagnosis.

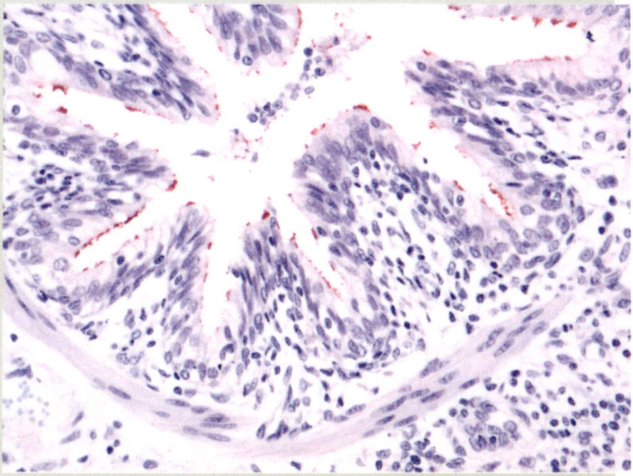

Figure 3. Positive immunoreaction (brown colouration) indicating the presence of *M. hyopneumoniae* antigen in the respiratory epithelial cilia of the bronchi in an infected pig. IHC. Magnification of the original image: 400×. Image courtesy of Dr Marisa Andrada (University of Las Palmas de Gran Canaria, Spain).

DETECTING GENETIC MATERIAL

In situ hybridisation (ISH) is a histological technique based on the ability of the genetic material to hybridise, i.e. bind completely to another strand of nucleic acid. In this case, DNA that complements a fragment of *M. hyopneumoniae* DNA (a hybridisation probe) is used. As is the case with antibodies, the hybridisation probe is labelled with a substance that, if the target DNA is present, can be visualised. The limitations of this technique are similar to those of IHC and IF, but it is more specific. Again, only specialised laboratories have refined this type of technique, so its use is mainly limited to research.

The main advantage of IHC, IF and ISH is that they allow a correlation between the presence of *M. hyopneumoniae* and the lung lesions observed to be established.

There is still no a reference technique to diagnose *M. hyopneumoniae* infection, but polymerase chain reaction (PCR) is currently the most commonly used technique. There are many tests available, and they are used routinely in most veterinary diagnostic laboratories. This technique also has various advantages:

- Can be used ante and postmortem, as it can be run on a variety of sample types.
- High level of sensitivity and specificity.
- Can be used on a large scale, enabling a useful number of samples to be processed at the same time.
- Very good for rapid diagnosis.

However, the technique also has limitations:

- High risk of contamination.
- Detects DNA from dead bacteria as well as live ones, so identifying a positive animal by PCR does not necessarily imply an active infection.

The development of different tests based on PCR has provided a direct method of detecting *M. hyopneumoniae* nucleic acids. PCR is a sensitive and specific method that can be applied to a wide range of samples. PCR tests can potentially detect the pathogen in the first stages of the disease, even before a detectable immune response has developed and/or there are any clinical signs.

Detection of *M. hyopneumoniae* by PCR determines the moment of infection more precisely than the time taken to seroconvert, which can vary considerably with *M. hyopneumoniae*.

Three different types of PCR are mainly used to detect *M. hyopneumoniae* (Table 4).

Table 4. **Main types of PCR used to detect *M. hyopneumoniae*.**

Type of PCR	Advantages	Disadvantages
Conventional	• Economical	• Lower sensitivity
Nested	• High sensitivity	• High risk of contamination (false positives) • Longer and more laborious procedure
Real-time or quantitative	• Enables DNA to be quantified • Quick • Low risk of contamination	• More expensive

DETECTING SPECIFIC ANTIBODIES

Serological testing to detect specific antibodies continues to be the most common way to detect exposure to *M. hyopneumoniae*. ELISA (enzyme-linked immunosorbent assay) is the most common test used, although there are other techniques to detect antibodies, such as the complement fixation test. ELISA is quick and economical, and can be automated, so it tends to be the most useful serological technique for herd monitoring. However, ELISA does have some significant limitations which must be taken into account if results are to be interpreted correctly. These are:

- Variable results depending on the commercial kit used, even when run on the same sample.
- Specificity can be affected by cross-reaction between the antibodies used and other mycoplasmas, especially *M. flocculare*.
- Impossible to differentiate between maternal antibodies, antibodies generated in response to infection, or antibodies resulting from vaccination.

- Time taken to seroconvert after infection is variable, so it is difficult to infer the timing of infection from the moment of seroconversion.
- No correlation between the level of serum antibodies (from infection or vaccination) and the level of protection against the disease.

Although PCR will confirm the presence of *M. hyopneumoniae*, the use of serological tests to assess antibody levels continues to be the most common method of detecting exposure to the pathogen.

Most commercial ELISA kits to detect *M. hyopneumoniae* are indirect, although some use competitive techniques (Fig. 4).

The sensitivity of techniques to diagnose *M. hyopneumoniae*, either by direct or indirect detection, can be affected by the genetic variability of the pathogen, i.e. by the existence of different strains. However, there is only considered to be one *M. hyopneumoniae* serotype.

Figure 4. Graphic representation of the indirect and competitive ELISA techniques used to detect antibodies to *M. hyopneumoniae*. With indirect ELISA, the intensity of the colour in the well is **directly** proportional to the level of specific antibodies in the serum but, with the competitive technique, this intensity is **indirectly** proportional to this antibody level.

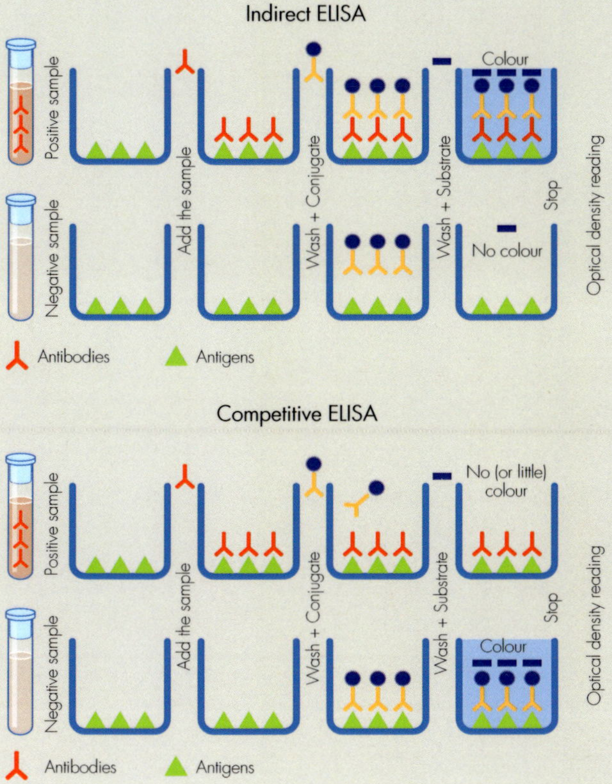

SAMPLING

Some potential diagnostic scenarios are described below:

The type of sample to be analysed depends on the clinical circumstances of the farm or herd, on the purpose (disease diagnosis, serological monitoring or detection of the pathogen), and on the diagnostic technique to be used.

SUSPICION OF AN EPIDEMIC FORM

If an acute outbreak of EP is suspected on a previously negative farm (i.e. an epidemic form), it is advisable to examine the lungs and use one of the aetiological diagnostic tools, such as PCR.

Necropsy and/or inspection at the abattoir

Necropsy of clinically affected pigs and/or lung inspection at the abattoir:

- Enables detection of CVPC.
- Allows collection of samples from the lower respiratory tract (Table 5).

Table 5. Postmortem samples for aetiological diagnosis of EP.

What samples can be taken?	How should they be transported?	Which techniques can be used?
Lung tissue	Refrigerated	Bacterial culture PCR
	Frozen	IF
	Formalin	Histopathology IHC ISH
BALF[1]	Refrigerated	Bacterial culture PCR
Bronchial swabs	Refrigerated	PCR

[1]Bronchoalveolar lavage fluid.

It is important to include the area of interface between the damaged and healthy lung tissue for laboratory testing, as this is where most viable organisms tend to be concentrated.

Sampling and PCR

In the event of an epidemic outbreak, clinically affected pigs should be sampled to detect *M. hyopneumoniae* by PCR. A range of samples can be taken for this purpose (Table 6); nasal swabs are the most common and easy to take, although they are not the most sensitive for detecting the pathogen.

Ideally, an in vivo sample that is used to detect a pathogen should be quick and easy to take. In this sense, oral fluid samples appear to be promising (Fig. 6). However, experimental results have been inconsistent, so such samples are not a very reliable source to assess the *M. hyopneumoniae* infection status. Laryngeal or tracheal swabs, or tracheobronchial lavage fluid (TBLF) have proven significantly more sensitive than nasal swabs in experimental and natural infections. TBLF and tracheal swabs are not very practical, so laryngeal swabs represent a new method with the potential for early diagnosis of

Table 6. Ante mortem samples for aetiological diagnosis of EP.

What samples can be taken?	How should they be transported?	Practicality	Sensitivity
Nasal swabs	All these samples should be refrigerated during transport	green	yellow
Laryngeal swabs		yellow	green
Tracheal swabs		red	green
TBLF[1]		red	green
Oral fluids		green	red

[1]Tracheobronchial lavage fluid.

Legend: green: very good; yellow: good; red: moderate.

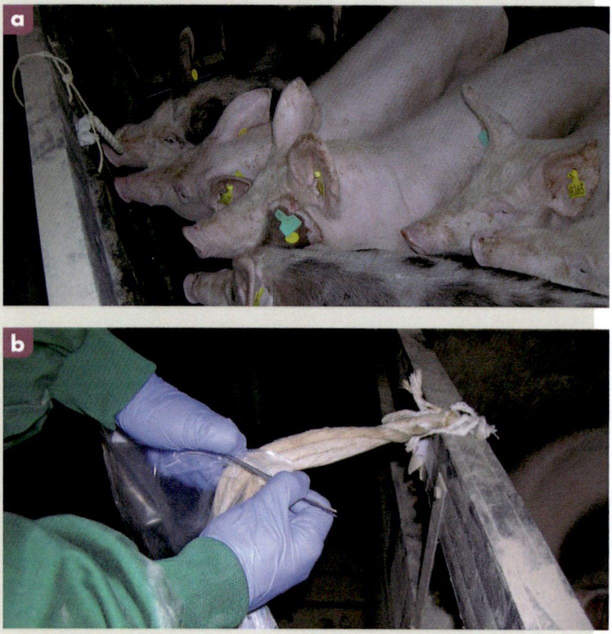

Figure 5. Placement of sampling rope in pen (a) and collecting oral fluids (b) in a pig herd. Image courtesy of Dr Elisa Gibert (Autonomous University of Barcelona, Spain).

M. hyopneumoniae infection, even in situations where exposure is suspected in the absence of clinical signs.

Laryngeal swabs tested by PCR are particularly practical and reliable diagnostic samples for in vivo detection of *M. hyopneumoniae*, especially in the early stages of infection.

In a vaccinated herd, it would be wrong to base *M. hyopneumoniae* infection status on serological results only, as antibodies from infection cannot be distinguished from vaccine-elicited antibodies. In these cases, it is especially advisable to combine serology with another technique, such as PCR.

MONITORING *M. HYOPNEUMONIAE* INFECTION STATUS ON A FARM (ENDEMIC FORM)

Serology is of limited use in acute cases, due to the period that elapses between infection and the ability to detect antibodies in the blood (seroconversion). However, for monitoring a farm that is endemically infected with *M. hyopneumoniae*, taking blood samples for ELISA is the most useful method. In general, two types of serological profiles (or antibody profiles) can be obtained on farm:

- **Cross-sectional antibody profile.** Samples are taken only once, simultaneously testing groups of animals of different ages and stages of production from the same herd. This type of sampling provides information on the health status of the farm with respect to a particular pathogen at a particular moment. However, when interpreting the results it is important to remember that the animals tested in each age group are individuals that can represent different situations, for example, vaccinated or unvaccinated, or with maternal antibodies.
- **Longitudinal antibody profile.** This is used to monitor a group of animals throughout their production cycle. This type of study allows the antibody response of a particular group of animals to be determined, and extrapolated to give an overall antibody profile of the farm. Although this type of profile provides very useful information, it is less widely used because it requires animals to be identified and monitored throughout the production cycle.

One of the greatest advantages of cross-sectional serological sampling over longitudinal sampling is the rapid availability of results.

MONITORING TO CONFIRM NEGATIVE STATUS

Many pig producers and genetics companies choose to eliminate *M. hyopneumoniae* as the best long-term strategy to control the infection. In these cases, confirmation of negative status by monitoring healthy pigs on the farm is essential and can be achieved by screening a representative number of pigs in high-risk age groups (i.e. fattening) for *M. hyopneumoniae* infection. The most effective combination for this purpose is considered to be PCR, ideally run on laryngeal swabs, and blood sampling for antibody detection. These tests should be performed regularly and be accompanied by periodic lung examinations at the abattoir.

3

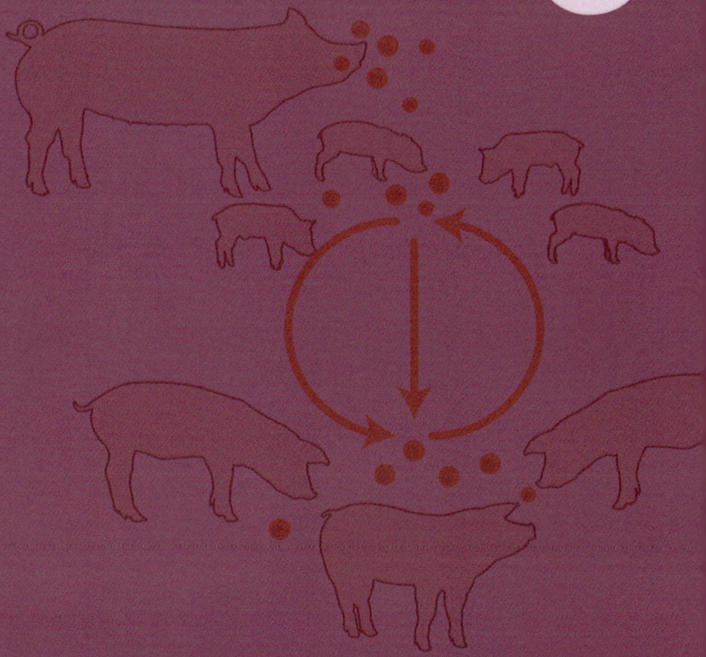

HOW AND WHEN IS *M. HYOPNEUMONIAE* TRANSMITTED?

DISTRIBUTION AND PREVALENCE

M. hyopneumoniae is found worldwide, and is a major concern for most countries that have intensive pig farming systems. Although farms that are free of *M. hyopneumoniae* may be found in many countries, the infection is endemic in a large proportion of farms. Prevalence is low in countries like Denmark, Finland, Sweden and Switzerland, which all run local eradication programmes, or have done so in the past. There is no specific or official information on the prevalence of *M. hyopneumoniae* in most countries, basically because EP is not a notifiable disease (except in Switzerland). Table 1 summarises the epidemiological data on EP and *M. hyopneumoniae* in different countries.

Table 1. Epidemiological data on EP in various countries (to 2014).

Country	Sampling year	No. of herds assessed	No. of lungs assessed	Prevalence of CVPC
Denmark	1994–1995	8	830	38.8 %
Spain	2002–04	39	1,365	8.4 %
	2007	107	10,404	55.7 %
Italy	2004–05	109	10,041	59.6 %
	2008	48	4,889	46.4 %
The Netherlands	2005–06	10	968	38 %
United Kingdom	2005–12	46,321	2,061,779	27.1 %
France	2006–08	125	3,750	69.3 %
Belgium	2007	60	6,335	23.9 %
	2012–13	30	3,820	25.9 %
Germany	2011–12	20	854	55.9 %
Sweden	–	4	1,600	3.3 %
China	2014	–	155	18.7 %

[1]Percentage of herds with at least one seropositive animal.
[2]Vaccinated against *M. hyopneumoniae*.
[3]Study of pigs farmed in semi-intensive conditions.

Although it is during the fattening and finishing periods that the number of infected pigs is high and signs of disease may be evident, infection can occur at any stage of production. The prevalence of *M. hyopneumoniae* in animals at different stages of production is shown in Table 2 (data published since 2000).

EP is widespread throughout the pig population and is endemic on most farms worldwide. It can affect animals of all ages, but it is uncommon in animals younger than 6 weeks of age.

Seropositive herds[1]	Average seropositivity of each herd	Percentage of vaccinated farms[2]	Source
100 %	85.9 %	-	Andreasen et al. (2001)
89.7 %	43.4 %	23.1 %	Martínez et al. (2009)
82 %	-	≥42 %	Fraile et al. (2010)
-	-	≥44 %	Ostanello et al. (2007)
100 %	-	79 %	Merialdi et al. (2012)
-	-	-	Jirawattanapong et al. (2010)
-	-	-	Eze et al. (2015)
93.6 %	70.8 %	92 %	Fablet et al. (2012)
98.3 %	79 %	≥80 %	Meyns et al. (2011)
100 %	74 %	100 %	Michiels et al. (2017)
-	-	100 %	Hillen et al. (2014)
-	-	0 %	Wallgren et al. (2016)
-	20.5 %	0 %	Qui et al. (2017)[3]

Table 2. Prevalence of *M. hyopneumoniae* by PCR on various samples, production stages and countries.

Production stage	Country	Nasal swabs	Laryngeal, bronchial or tracheal swabs
Suckling	Spain	0.0–6.4 %	0.0–5.4 %
		0.5–5.5 %	0.0–8.0 %
		5.0 %	-
	United States	0.0–51.3 %	-
		0.0–56.0 %	-
		-	0–2.5 %
	Germany	-	-
		-	-
		18.7 %	-
		3.6 %	-
	Hungary	10.0 %	-
	Poland	9.7 %	-
	Italy	22.1 %	-
	The Netherlands	7.7 %	-
	Brazil	-	0.0 %
Nursery pigs	Spain	2.0–9.0 %	0.0–8.0 %
	Germany	-	1.2 %
	Belgium and the Netherlands	-	-
Fatteners	Spain	21.8–61.1 %	42.0–86.0 %
	United States	-	8.0–100 %
Sows (including gilts)	Spain	24.0–56.0 %	-
	Germany	6.3–22.3 %	-
	Brazil	-	0.0–36.4 %
		-	0.0–67.4 %

[1]Tracheobronchial lavage fluid;
[2]Bronchoalveolar lavage fluid.

TBLF[1]	BALF[2]	Lung tissue	Reference
-	-	-	Sibila et al. (2007a)
-	-	-	Sibila et al. (2007b)
-	-	-	Villarreal et al. (2010)
-	-	-	Fano et al. (2007)
-	-	-	Pieters et al. (2014)
-	-	-	Vangroenweghe et al. (2015b)
-	12.3 %	-	Moorkamp et al. (2009)
-	-	2.0 %	Nathues et al. (2010)
-	-	-	Villarreal et al. (2010)
-	-	-	Nathues et al. (2013)
-	-	-	Villarreal et al. (2010)
-	-	-	Villarreal et al. (2010)
-	-	-	Villarreal et al. (2010)
-	-	-	Villarreal et al. (2010)
-	-	-	Takeuti et al. (2017a)
-	-	-	Sibila et al. (2007b)
-	-	-	Nathues et al. (2013b)
1.6–15.5 %	-	-	Vangroenweghe et al. (2015a)
-	-	-	Sibila et al. (2007b)
-	-	-	Fano et al. (2007)
-	-	-	Calsamiglia et al. (2000)
-	-	-	Nathues et al. (2013)
-	-	-	Takeuti et al. (2017a)
-	-	-	Takeuti et al. (2017b)

M. HYOPNEUMONIAE: MODE AND TIMING OF TRANSMISSION

Although the disease can be introduced by airborne transmission, the most common source of *M. hyopneumoniae* infection is direct contact with respiratory tract secretions from infected pigs. In this way, infected pigs entering a farm introduce the organism into the premises or herd by direct transmission. Once on the farm, infection is maintained by direct contact, both vertically from the sow to her piglets, and horizontally between animals in the same pen (Fig. 1).

Figure 1. Diagram of *M. hyopneumoniae* transmission routes.

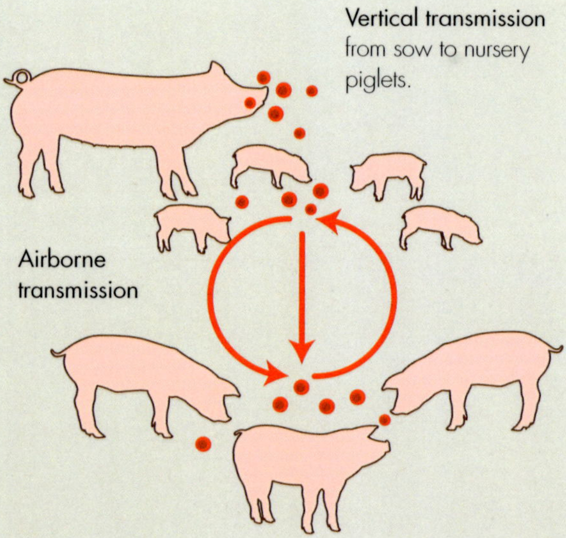

Experimentally, *M. hyopneumoniae* has been found to spread for a distance of 9.2 km by airborne transmission.

Vectors do not seem to play a significant role in *M. hyopneumoniae* transmission.

Piglets are considered to be free of infection at birth and are first exposed to the pathogen through contact with the dam when suckling. Therefore, the infection status of the sow during the suckling period determines the degree of *M. hyopneumoniae* colonisation of the piglet at weaning. This degree of colonisation may have an effect on the subsequent clinical presentation and severity of the disease. Sows are considered to be crucial to the persistence of *M. hyopneumoniae* infection as they transmit the infection not only to their progeny, but also to newly introduced gilts, perpetuating the infection on the farm.

It has been suggested that longer suckling periods could increase the risk of *M. hyopneumoniae* colonisation of the piglet.

Young and low-parity sows are thought to be the main source of infection for piglets, as they are probably at an earlier stage of infection, and therefore excrete more bacteria than older sows. The constant addition of replacement gilts and birth of new piglets provide susceptible populations that keep spreading *M. hyopneumoniae* within the herd or farm.

Good gilt acclimatisation can reduce the risk of *M. hyopneumoniae* infection in their piglets, reducing the likelihood of them developing clinical signs of EP during fattening.

Very long–lasting *M. hyopneumoniae* infection has been described in some individuals, and these animals can continue to excrete the bacteria, and even spread infection, for as long as 214 days p.i. However, the duration and kinetics of this excretion are difficult to determine, and it is not known whether excretion is uniform and continuous, or variable and intermittent. The organism's persistence and its ability to create asymptomatic carriers are particularly important factors for animals that remain on the farm for any length of time, as is the case for breeding sows. The slow transmission of *M. hyopneumoniae* complicates understanding of the infection in this group of animals even further. One study determined that introducing one infected sow to a group infects only approximately 0.77 susceptible sows after one week of exposure.

The critical features of *M. hyopneumoniae* epidemiology are its persistence and infectivity.

DYNAMICS OF *M. HYOPNEUMONIAE* INFECTION

Under experimental conditions, pigs are usually negative for *M. hyopneumoniae* and they are then inoculated with higher doses of bacteria than under farm conditions. In some cases, lung lesions and coughing start to be seen as early as 7 days p.i., with the most severe lung lesions tending to be seen around 4 weeks p.i. However, *M. hyopneumoniae* antibody induction is slow and the time between infection and seroconversion is fairly variable. Seroconversion has been detected experimentally at 7 days p.i., but it is thought that it would take all the pigs in a group 7–9 weeks to seroconvert.

The incubation period is difficult to predict under natural conditions. The combination of serology and *M. hyopneumoniae* detection by PCR (respiratory tract swab or lavage) has provided a clearer understanding of the circulation and transmission of these bacteria in individual batches and throughout the entire farm. Patterns of infection and seroconversion are different for each farm or batch, indicating that the dynamics of *M. hyopneumoniae* infection are very variable and depend on various factors that affect infection pressure. Each farm should therefore be considered an individual case, and extrapolation is risky when designing a control or prevention programme.

The factors that affect the dynamics of *M. hyopneumoniae* infection are:

- Production system.
- Management practices.
- Housing and weather conditions.
- Concomitant or secondary infections.
- Immune status of the animal.
- Strain of *M. hyopneumoniae*.

4

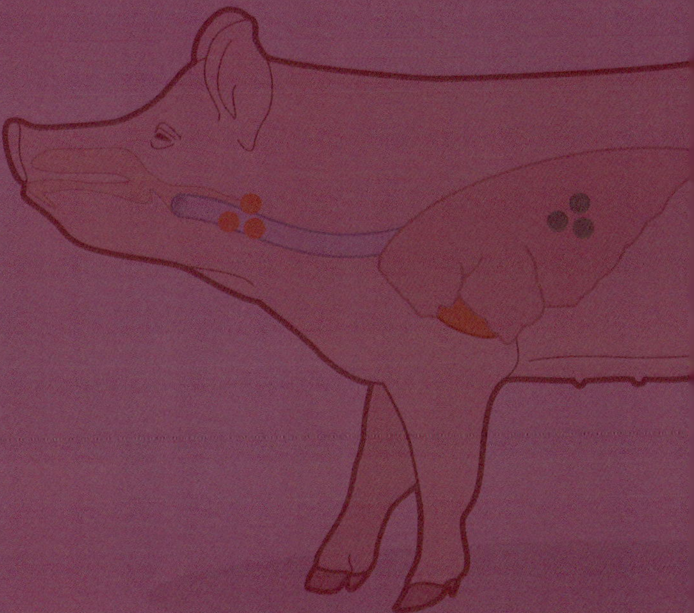

WHAT DO WE KNOW ABOUT *M. HYOPNEUMONIAE* STRAINS?

Various strains of *M. hyopneumoniae* that differ in their genome and virulence have been discovered so far, but the implications and actual effects of this are still largely unknown.

Importantly, in order for control measures to be more effective, a better understanding is needed on the variability between different strains of *M. hyopneumoniae*, and how this variability has an impact on the epidemiology of the disease.

DIVERSITY OF *M. HYOPNEUMONIAE*

The dynamics of infection differ considerably under field conditions, and this leads to much variation in the clinical signs and lung lesions associated with enzootic pneumonia (EP). This variability has been attributed to factors such as coinfection, management, housing and environmental conditions, and to the fact that strains of *M. hyopneumoniae* may vary in virulence. The latter has promoted the detection and genetic characterisation of *M. hyopneumoniae* isolates as a main objective for epidemiological studies. As a result, more information has been discovered about the diversity of *M. hyopneumoniae* strains.

M. hyopneumoniae strains are known to be genetically heterogeneous, but it is not yet clear whether there is an association between genetic variation and virulence.

Genotyping techniques have enabled *M. hyopneumoniae* strains to be differentiated genetically. Despite their overall genetic homogeneity, various DNA regions do vary, and are thus termed polymorphic. These are the regions that are analysed using genotyping techniques, and they are used to detect subpopulations (strains) of *M. hyopneumoniae*. One of the techniques that is most commonly used for this pathogen analyses paired clusters of gene sequences at specific loci called variable number tandem repeats (VNTR). More than one of these gene sequences is usually analysed, as shown in Fig. 1, where three loci are examined using multiple loci VNTR analysis (MLVA).

VARIABILITY FROM COUNTRY TO COUNTRY OR REGION TO REGION

Different *M. hyopneumoniae* strains have been detected in different countries, and on different farms in a particular region. However, there are reports of regions or neighbouring farms where only one strain, or very similar strains, are in circulation. Overall results may seem slightly contradictory, but they depend to a certain extent on the accuracy of the genotyping technique used. No particular *M. hyopneumoniae* strain has yet been associated with a particular country or geographical region. It has been suggested that the proximity of farms and the mixing of animals of different origins could introduce new *M. hyopneumoniae* strains, increasing diversity. This means that *M. hyopneumoniae* strains are likely to be more heterogeneous in areas of intensive production and/or where there is significant trading of pigs (Fig. 2).

Figure 1. Diagram explaining the MLVA technique.

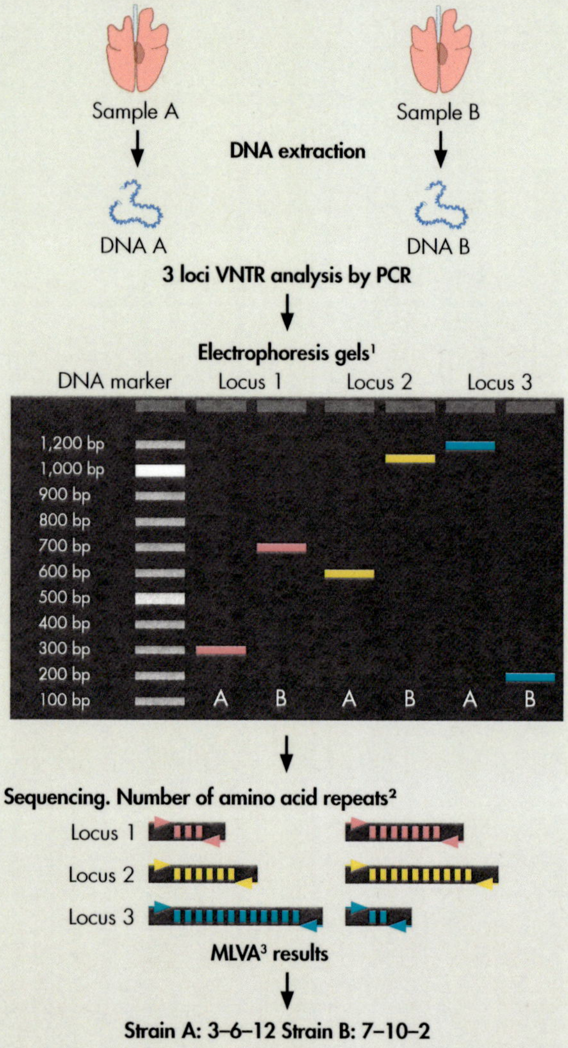

[1]The three DNA regions amplified (loci 1, 2 and 3) have different molecular weights in samples A and B.

[2]The number of amino acid repeats can be inferred from the size of these fragments. If sequencing is used, the repeats can be counted accurately.

[3]Each strain is defined by the number of repeats at each of the loci analysed.

Figure 2. Diagram of a hypothetical situation with various *M. hyopneumoniae* strains (coloured circles) in an area with low production density, and another with high density.

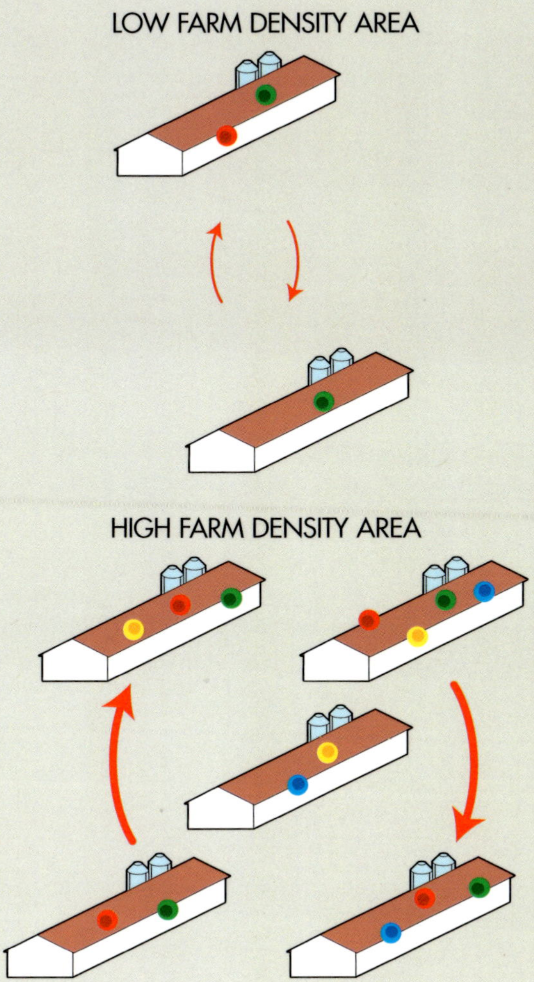

VARIABILITY ON AN INDIVIDUAL FARM

More than one strain of the pathogen can be found on a farm or in a herd, even when animals are vaccinated against *M. hyopneumoniae*. The *M. hyopneumoniae* transmission cycle can be interrupted in all-in/all-out production systems, so it has been suggested that there could be less variability in the *M. hyopneumoniae* strains circulating on farms that follow this production system than on farms with continuous production, where it seems to be easier to introduce new strains and for them to persist.

> Up to 13 different strains of *M. hyopneumoniae* have been detected in one batch of pigs.

VARIABILITY BETWEEN PIGS

One individual can be affected by multiple strains of *M. hyopneumoniae*. This heterogeneity has been observed both in cases of infection by *M. hyopneumoniae* alone, and where there is coinfection with other pig pathogens. Different strains have also been detected in the same anatomical location (e.g. the lung) in an individual, and in different locations (e.g. the lung and trachea) in the same animal (Fig. 3).

> Up to 3 different strains of *M. hyopneumoniae* have been found in one single animal.

HOW DOES THE DIVERSITY OF STRAINS AFFECT CLINICAL PRESENTATION?

Experimentally, *M. hyopneumoniae* strains have been classified into high- and low-virulence strains: the distinguishing

Figure 3. Diagram of the respiratory organs of the pig, showing the different *M. hyopneumoniae* strains that have been detected in a single individual so far.

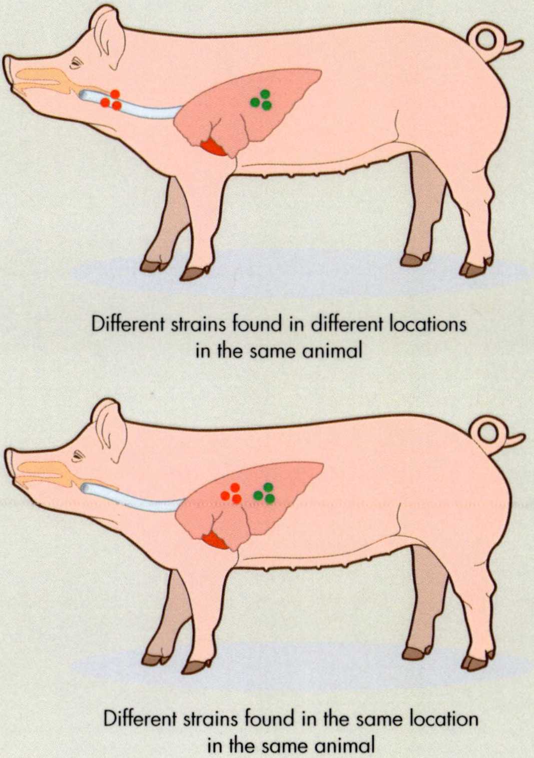

features of both types are summarised in Table 1. On farms, the effect of *M. hyopneumoniae* variability on the severity of lung lesions and its effect on the onset and duration of clinical signs has yet to be clearly defined. Some studies have indicated that coinfection by more than one strain results in more severe lung lesions, but this additive effect has not been confirmed by other studies.

Currently, the lack of a known genetic marker for virulence, combined with the existence of different strains, makes it difficult to understand the effect of strain variability on clinical presentation, both at an individual and farm level.

The existence of different strains of the pathogen could have significant repercussions on the efficacy of control and prevention methods (vaccination and/or antibiotic treatment), and on the sensitivity of diagnostic techniques. However, these aspects are still largely unknown.

The importance of *M. hyopneumoniae* variability and the implications for the pig sector are still to be determined.

EFFECT OF VARIABILITY ON VACCINE EFFICACY

Antigenic differences between *M. hyopneumoniae* strains have been reported, and this could mean that the antibody profile generated by a vaccine strain may not be exactly the same as that generated by circulating field strains. This would suggest that the degree of protection provided by a vaccine could partly depend on its similarity to the infection strain. Despite this, an experimental study compared the protection offered by a homologous vaccine (vaccine strain identical to the inoculation strain) and a heterologous vaccine (vaccine strain different from the inoculation strain). No conclusive differences were found regarding the level of protection conferred.

The fact that the most virulent strains can be more immunogenic (Table 1) could have consequences for vaccination. One trial using a commercial vaccine suggested it was more effective in animals challenged with a high virulence strain than in those

Table 1. The distinguishing characteristics of high and low virulence strains of *M. hyopneumoniae* have been described in various experimental studies.

	High virulence strains	Low virulence strains
Clinical signs	More pronounced cough and earlier onset of clinical signs	No cough. When there is cough, it is less severe and starts later
Production parameters	Variable effect on daily weight gain	Unaffected in most cases
Lung lesions	More animals affected. Lesions are more severe	Fewer animals affected. Lesions are less severe
Seroconversion	*M. hyopneumoniae* antibodies usually appear at an early stage (seroconversion closer to infection)	*M. hyopneumoniae* antibodies usually appear at a later stage (seroconversion further from infection)
Immunogenicity	Stronger proinflammatory effect, with more cytokine production and inflammatory cell infiltration at a local level	Weaker proinflammatory response
Multiplication	Higher multiplication rate. Possible dissemination to other internal organs	Lower multiplication rate. Dissemination to other internal organs not reported
Transmission	No significant differences	
Adhesion	No significant differences	
Adaptation to in vitro culture medium	Expression of more proteins related to adhesion and colonisation of the pig's respiratory tract	Expression of more proteins related to metabolism and growth

Beatriz García-Morante, Joaquim Segalés and Marina Sibila, SUIS no. 115, 2015.

challenged with a low virulence strain. The comparison was made with a non-vaccinated control group. This could be because highly virulent strains induce a more severe inflammatory response (and therefore lesions), and thus would be more likely to show a greater difference from the control group. Another trial also demonstrated the efficacy of a commercial vaccine against coinfection with two different *M. hyopneumoniae* strains, one of high virulence and the other of low virulence.

EFFECT OF VARIABILITY ON ANTIBIOTIC EFFICACY

Other studies have discovered in vitro acquisition of resistance by various field strains of *M. hyopneumoniae* especially to fluoroquinolones, but also to macrolides and lincosamides. This highlights the fact that there may be different strains of *M. hyopneumoniae*, with varying antibiotic sensitivity, on the same farm. Information on the relationship between genetic variability and a predisposition to develop antibiotic resistance is very scarce. One single article, however, demonstrated that resistance to macrolides and lincosamides could be caused by mutations that affect the 23S ribosomal RNA (a component of the 50S subunit of the prokaryotic ribosome). This has also been described in other *Mycoplasma* species.

EFFECT OF VARIABILITY ON SENSITIVITY OF DIAGNOSTIC TECHNIQUES

Genetic differences between *M. hyopneumoniae* strains have been reported to give rise to false negatives with some diagnostic techniques, such as PCR. Although there is currently a wide range of PCR-based techniques to detect the DNA of *M. hyopneumoniae* in various sample types, no single PCR has been established as the reference test. It is not known whether the degree of colour change in serological tests like ELISA is modified by the antibody profile generated by a particular strain. However, highly virulent strains are generally assumed to induce a quicker specific antibody response (Table 1).

5

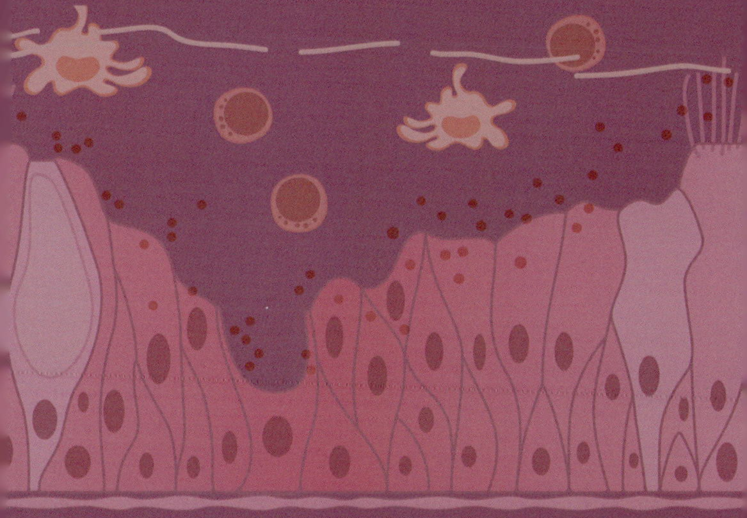

WHAT HAPPENS AFTER INFECTION?

DISEASE RISK FACTORS

Enzootic pneumonia (EP) onset and severity are affected by various factors (Fig. 1) and it is important to understand these in order to control the disease. Various risk factors have been described at an individual and farm level that seem to increase the probability of animals being infected and going on to develop EP (Table 1).

> The risk factors identified for *M. hyopneumoniae* infection highlight that the approach to prevent and control EP must be multifactorial and tailored to each individual farm.

Figure 1. Factors potentially affecting the onset and severity of EP in pigs.

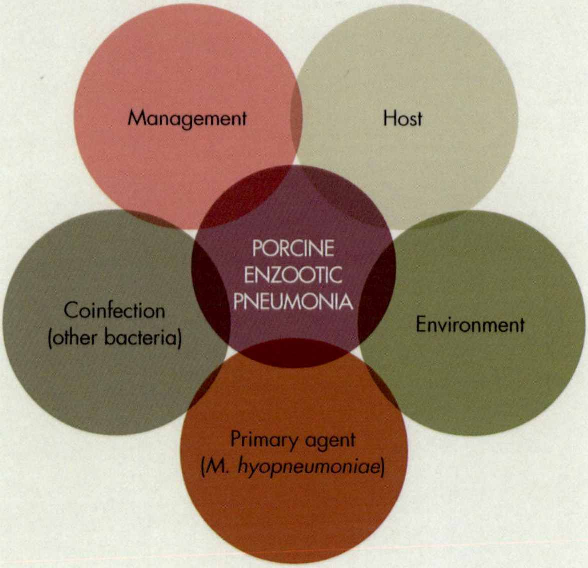

Table 1. Potential risk factors for *M. hyopneumoniae* infection described in the literature.

Risk factor	Definition
Weather conditions	• High rainfall. • Low temperatures.
Geographical location of the farm	• Proximity to other pig farms. • Proximity to a road.
Production system	• Continuous flow.
Repopulation policy	• Frequent entry of replacement gilts (>120/year). • Poor acclimatisation of gilts and boars. • No vaccination against *M. hyopneumoniae* during acclimatisation.
Housing	• High pen stocking rate. • High number of pens per barn in farrowing accommodation (>16 pens).
Sow parity	• First or second gestation.
Management during breeding stage	• High fostering rate. • Long lactation period. • Low temperatures in piglet bedding area. • Piglet teeth not clipped/ground. • Piglets only given one dose of iron.
Weaning management strategy	• No vaccination against *M. hyopneumoniae*.

The greatest risk for introducing *M. hyopneumoniae* into a farm that is negative for the pathogen is the entry of infected animals.

Once these critical factors are known, the likelihood of pathogen transmission and infection can be reduced. In endemic situations, piglets infected by *M. hyopneumoniae* are considered to be the initiators that spread the disease. Identifying risk factors during the suckling period could help create intervention strategies to prevent *M. hyopneumoniae* transmission from sows to their progeny and, therefore reduce the effect of the disease in fattening units.

Close correlation between colonisation with *M. hyopneumoniae* at weaning and the subsequent onset, and even severity, of EP in fattening pigs has been seen in some studies. Therefore, reducing or eliminating risk factors during the lactation period could help reduce the incidence of *M. hyopneumoniae* infection in the piglet and probably the prevalence of EP in subsequent stages.

MANAGEMENT, HOUSING AND BIOSECURITY

Improving management practices is essential to control *M. hyopneumoniae* infection. Implementing management changes to reduce the potential of infection by *M. hyopneumoniae* can improve EP control considerably. The main action points are discussed below.

PRODUCTION SYSTEM

In continuous flow production systems, as soon as individual pigs are regrouped to be transferred to the next production stage, they are mixed with animals of different ages. This is a source of stress and increases the potential for pathogen transmission and infection. Conversely, in all-in/all-out systems the transmission cycles for many pathogens between animals of different ages are interrupted. These systems also allow environmental conditions to be tailored to a uniform population of animals, and facilities can be cleaned after emptying. Clearly, the practice of mixing animals from different sources increases the likelihood of disease, even in all-in/all-out systems.

GILT ACCLIMATISATION

Improving herd genetics has encouraged the introduction of new animals into the herd and the risk of disrupting herd immunity increases when this replacement rate is high. In these cases, it is important to assess the health status of the farm of origin, especially their gilts, and try to ensure that it is at least as good as the receiving farm. Gilts must also be properly acclimatised.

> Good gilt acclimatisation is essential for effective management of *M. hyopneumoniae* infection on farm.

Effective gilt acclimatisation should ideally reduce *M. hyopneumoniae* excretion at first farrowing, resulting in lower piglet colonisation by weaning, which may then lead to fewer respiratory problems during the fattening stage. A survey published in Europe in 2017 revealed that vaccination against *M. hyopneumoniae* is the most commonly used acclimatisation procedure, followed by vaccination combined with exposure to selected animals (usually culled sows).

STOCKING DENSITY

Reducing stocking rate during the various production stages reduces the incidence of respiratory disease.

> High densities increase pathogen transmission.

BIOSECURITY

No specific biosecurity measures have been developed to prevent and/or control *M. hyopneumoniae* infection, but it is advisable to implement general biosecurity strategies, maintain a "disease-free" status, and prevent new strains being introduced. *M. hyopneumoniae* does not seem to be spread in any significant way by fomites, and programmes of regular cleaning and disinfection are effective against this pathogen. *M. hyopneumoniae* survival outside the host has always been thought to be limited, although one study suggests that it can survive on some plastic surfaces and in dust for up to 8 days at low temperatures (4 °C).

DURATION OF THE LACTATION PERIOD

Early weaning (<3 weeks) can reduce *M. hyopneumoniae* transmission from the sow to her progeny. However, weaning is one of the most critical stages of pig production and causes significant physiological stress to the piglet. Therefore, early weaning is not routinely practised in Europe, despite its success in reducing piglet colonisation by *M. hyopneumoniae* and other pathogens.

The longer the lactation period, the greater the risk of piglets being colonised by *M. hyopneumoniae*. However, the lactation period cannot be reduced indiscriminately, as other factors have to be considered (legislation, management, facilities, etc.).

FOSTERING

Piglet viability in the first few days of life depends to a great extent on the level of passive immunity acquired through the colostrum. Antibodies and immune cells are transferred to the piglet in different ways: antibodies are absorbed by the intestinal mucosa, regardless of the maternal source, but lymphocytes have to be viable and must have been produced by the piglet's biological mother. Piglets raised by a foster sow from the first day of life could therefore be potentially deficient in the specific cell-mediated immune response to infectious agents, including *M. hyopneumoniae*. Therefore, fostering should be minimised wherever possible, and it should be carried out all at once, after having first allowed all the piglets to have suckled their biological mothers.

ANTIMICROBIAL THERAPY

The most common antibiotics to control and treat respiratory diseases, including *M. hyopneumoniae* infection, are: tetracyclines, macrolides, lincosamides, pleuromutilins, fluoroquinolones, florfenicol, aminoglycosides and aminocyclitols. It is important to remember that this pathogen is intrinsically resistant to antibiotics that work by interference with polymerisation of bacterial cell wall precursors, such as the β-lactams. Resistance to other types of antibiotics does not seem to be a problem when treating *M. hyopneumoniae* infections. However, this may not be the case for the other bacteria often involved in EP. *M. hyopneumoniae* strains with different sensitivity to antimicrobials may coexist on the same farm, although this subject has not yet been examined in any depth.

> Aminoglycosides are effective against mycoplasmas, but oral absorption is limited and withdrawal times are excessively long when administered parenterally, so they are generally of little practical use against *M. hyopneumoniae*.

VACCINATION

Vaccination against *M. hyopneumoniae* is probably the strategy that is most widely used worldwide to control EP. Most commercial vaccines are bacterins, i.e., based on inactivated *M. hyopneumoniae* cells, combined with an adjuvant, and injected intramuscularly. Different commercial vaccine manufacturers use different strains of *M. hyopneumoniae* as a base for their vaccines. Table 2 provides an overview of the characteristics of the vaccines commercially available in Europe.

EP cannot be controlled by vaccination alone. An effective control programme should be based on a combination of different strategies that act at different levels.

As with antimicrobial treatments, vaccination usually reduces clinical signs and lung lesions, and prevents or reduces the effect on production parameters. Commercial vaccines also reduce the number of bacteria found in the respiratory tract and the prevalence of the infection. However, vaccination does not prevent colonisation entirely, and only slightly reduces *M. hyopneumoniae* transmission.

The exact mechanisms of vaccine protection are largely unknown. On the one hand, serum antibodies to *M. hyopneumoniae* generated by vaccination are not sufficient to evaluate either the effectiveness of the immune response, nor the degree of protection against the disease. On the other hand, although the importance of local antibodies in the respiratory mucosa is still unclear, a series of studies have been carried out that suggest that the cellular immune response is important for protection.

Vaccinating against *M. hyopneumoniae* can potentially reduce the effect of the disease, but it does not prevent colonisation of the animal or transmission of the pathogen.

The best age at vaccination for maximum benefit is still not entirely clear. Single and double vaccination strategies are both common methods for preventing *M. hyopneumoniae* infection. Animals are often vaccinated at 1 week of age, or at weaning. Vaccine response usually improves with age, as piglet immune function matures and levels of maternal antibodies wane. However, in the case of *M. hyopneumoniae*, some studies have demonstrated that commercial vaccines can be effective to induce an antibody response even in the presence of maternal antibodies. Maternal antibody levels in the piglet at vaccination are probably more important than piglet age itself. Finally, vaccination at stressful moments for the animal, such as weaning, has been questioned. In fact, some experimental and field trials have demonstrated that vaccinating piglets some days before weaning could give better results than vaccinating at weaning.

Optimising the moment of vaccination helps when designing and implementing more effective disease control programmes. A *M. hyopneumoniae* vaccination should aim to balance the advantages of late vaccination and the need to induce immunity before exposure to the pathogen.

Table 2. *M. hyopneumoniae* vaccines commercially available in Europe (source: Spanish Agency for Medicines and Medical Devices, 2018).

Vaccine	Strain	Adjuvant	Route of administration
HYOGEN®	2940	Light liquid paraffin and *Escherichia coli* J5 LPS	Intramuscular
Ingelvac MycoFLEX®	J (isolate B-3745)	Carbomer	Intramuscular
M+PAC™	J (ATCC[1] No. 25934)	Light mineral oil and aluminium hydroxide	Intramuscular
MYPRAVAC® SUIS	J	Levamisole hydrochloride and carbomer	Intramuscular
Porcilis® M Hyo	11	dl-α-tocopheryl acetate	Intramuscular
Porcilis® M Hyo ID Once	11	Light liquid paraffin and dl-α-tocopheryl acetate	Intramuscular
Porcilis® PCV M Hyo[2]	J	Light mineral oil and aluminium hydroxide	Intradermal
Rhinanvac® Pigs[3]	11	Aluminium hydroxide	Intramuscular
Stellamune™ Mycoplasma	NL1042	Amphigen® base (liquid paraffin and soya lecithin) and Drakeol® 5 (liquid paraffin)	Intramuscular
Stellamune™ ONE	NL1042	Amphigen® base (liquid paraffin and soya lecithin) and Drakeol® 5 (liquid paraffin)	Intramuscular
SUVAXYN® CIRCO+MH RTU[2]	P-5722-3	Squalene, poloxamer 401 and polysorbate 80	Intramuscular
SUVAXYN® M. hyo	P-5722-3	Carbomer	Intramuscular
SUVAXYN® MH-One	P-5722-3	Carbomer and squalene	Intramuscular

[1]American Type Culture Collection.

[2]Combined vaccine with PCV2.

[3]Combined vaccine with *B. bronchiseptica*, *H. parasuis*, *M. haemolytica* and *P. multocida* type D.

Age at administration	Booster	Onset and duration of immunity
≥21 days	No	Onset 3 weeks, duration 26 weeks following vaccination
≥21 days	No	Onset 2 weeks, duration 26 weeks following vaccination
≥7 days	No	Onset 4 weeks maximum, duration 24 weeks following vaccination
	Yes. If using 1 ml of product, doses 2–4 weeks apart	Onset 5 weeks, maximum duration 24 weeks after initial dose
≥7 days	Yes, 3 weeks later	Duration at least 10 weeks following vaccination
≥7 days	Yes, 3 weeks later	Onset 2 weeks, duration at least 20 weeks following second dose
≥7 days	No	Onset 3 weeks, duration 22 weeks following vaccination
≥14 days	No	Onset 4 weeks, duration 21 weeks following vaccination
=12 weeks	Yes, 3–4 weeks later	Onset 4 weeks, duration 24 weeks following second dose
≥7 days	Yes, 3–4 weeks later	Duration at least 22 weeks following second dose
≥3 days	No	Onset no later than 3 weeks, duration 26 weeks following vaccination
≥21 days	No	Onset 3 weeks, duration 23 weeks following vaccination
≥3 days	Yes, 2 weeks later	No information available
≥7 days	No	Onset 2 weeks, duration 24 weeks following vaccination

6

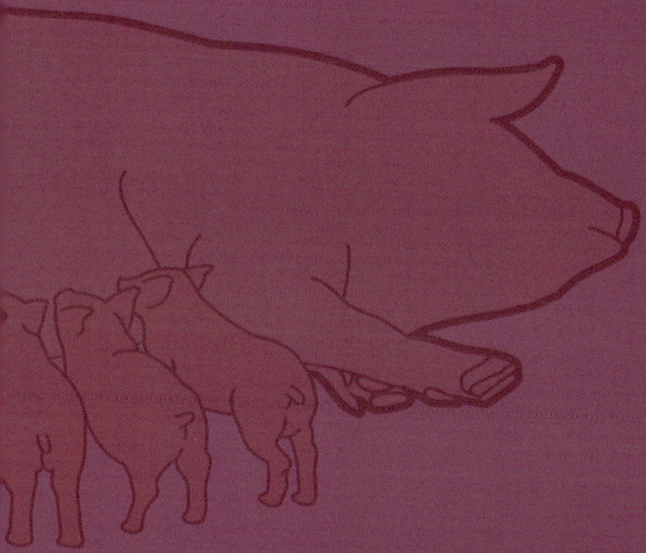

IS ERADICATION POSSIBLE?

JUSTIFICATION FOR ERADICATION PROGRAMMES

Mycoplasma hyopneumoniae continues to be one of the most prevalent and economically important respiratory pathogens in the pig industry. The financial cost of *M. hyopneumoniae* is probably the main reason why producers consider trying to eradicate it from their farms. Various *M. hyopneumoniae* eradication protocols have been described, and these are summarised in Table 1.

The losses associated with *M. hyopneumoniae*, and the creation of specific pathogen free (SPF) breeding stock for this pathogen, have led breeding farms to develop strategies to obtain and maintain negative herds.

ERADICATION PROGRAMMES

The most direct way of eradicating a pathogen and its associated diseases is total depopulation, followed by repopulation with individuals that are free from that particular pathogen. However, the high cost of this policy meant that initial efforts to eradicate *M. hyopneumoniae* were based on a more conservative method of partial depopulation followed by a subsequent pause in farrowing (the Swiss method). This method gained recognition in the 1990s, when Switzerland used it as their national plan to eradicate *M. hyopneumoniae* and *Actinobacillus pleuropneumoniae* infections. The Swiss method is based on the fact that *M. hyopneumoniae* persists on the farm because of the youngest animals (under 10 months of age), which are the main transmitters of infection to susceptible animals.

Small modifications have also been successfully introduced to the protocol in countries like Norway and Denmark. However, this strategy is of questionable efficacy on large farms, where there is a suspicion of the existence of subpopulations that are positive to the micro-organism, regardless of the age of the animals. Other protocols have been developed for these cases, such as herd closure (no admission of replacement gilts for a certain period) coupled with antibiotic medication, or medication alone. These are used to eradicate *M. hyopneumoniae* from weaned piglet producing farms.

In eradication protocols requiring herd closure and antibiotic medication, replacement gilts should not be brought into the herd for at least 8 months (240 days). This period is based on data that suggest that this length of time is the minimum required to ensure that animals have stopped shedding *M. hyopneumoniae* after infection. This means that replacement gilts brought onto the farm before closure should be acclimatised in a particular way (Fig. 1). This is considered critical for the programme to succeed.

Most swine breeder farms that supply replacements are currently free from *M. hyopneumoniae.* If one of these farms suffers an outbreak of EP, the standard procedure is to implement an eradication programme.

Figure 1. Time periods to be respected for *M. hyopneumoniae* negative replacement gilts in eradication programmes based on herd closure and antibiotic medication.

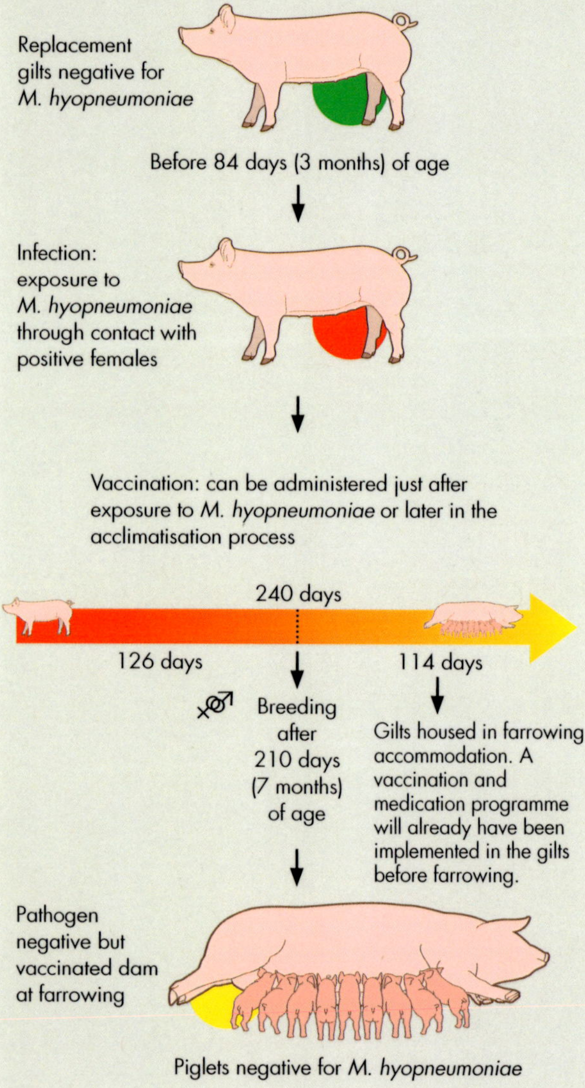

Table 1. Description, advantages and disadvantages of *M. hyopneumoniae* eradication programmes.

Eradication programme	Description	Advantages	Disadvantages
Depopulation-Repopulation	Removal of all the animals and repopulation with animals negative for *M. hyopneumoniae*.	• Higher success rate. • Potential to eradicate more than one pathogen/disease. • Potential to improve farm genetics.	• Very high cost due to total loss of production. • Impractical on farms with breeding animals of high genetic potential.
Partial depopulation (Swiss method)	Farm emptied of all animals under 10 months of age and farrowing paused for 2 weeks. All animals are medicated in this period.	• Relatively high success rate in the eradication programmes already implemented, in Switzerland for example.	• Questionable success on large farms. • High cost of emptying and treatment.
Closure and medication (modified Swiss method)	All females, including replacement gilts, exposed to *M. hyopneumoniae*. Once colonisation is proven, the farm is closed for at least 8 months. All animals are medicated and vaccinated against *M. hyopneumoniae* during this period. No pause in farrowing.	• Production losses minimised as no farrowing pause or removal of animals.	• High cost of antibiotic treatment and vaccination. • Risk of exposing sows to other pathogens.
Medication	Medication of the whole herd with a long-acting antibiotic (preferably injectable) against *M. hyopneumoniae*. Animals are usually treated twice, 2 weeks apart. Piglets born 4 weeks after the initial injection are also treated at birth and at 14 days of age.	• Quicker return to "*M. hyopneumoniae*-negative" status. • Less expensive procedure, as there is no loss of production.	• Lower success rate.

CONFIRMATION OF SUCCESSFUL ERADICATION

One of the most important features of any successful eradication programme is to ensure that the pathogen is not circulating in the population when the programme comes to an end. In the case of some pathogens, confirmation is easy, but it is more difficult to determine for *M. hyopneumoniae*, as doubts always remain as to whether the pathogen has been completely eradicated. If there are many cases where reinfection has occurred after implementation of an eradication programme, this will raise questions about that programme's actual efficacy. The introduction of this method in Switzerland has been acclaimed an overall success, as the incidence of EP has decreased dramatically, but it is worth noting that some sporadic cases have been detected in the last few years (3 cases were reported in 2016). Possible indirect *M. hyopneumoniae* infection should be borne in mind, as the bacteria are known to spread for considerable distances by airborne transmission (as far as 9.2 km has been reported) and maintain the potential to infect susceptible animals.

7

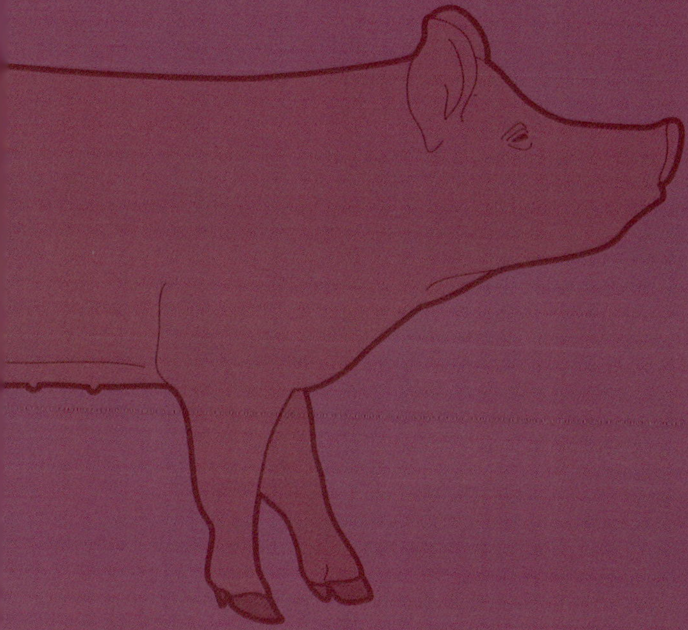

WHAT HAVE YOU LEARNT ABOUT THE DISEASE?

QUIZ

Now test yourself by answering the following questions. Only one answer is correct.

1. **Why are mycoplasmas resistant to β-lactam antibiotics like penicillin?**
   - **a.** They are Gram-positive micro-organisms (identified by Gram staining).
   - **b.** Their cell membranes contain sterols.
   - **c.** They lack cell walls.
   - **d.** They can metabolise this type of antibiotic.
2. **What is the immediate effect of *M. hyopneumoniae* colonisation of the upper respiratory tract?**
   - **a.** Dry nonproductive cough.
   - **b.** Ciliostasis and deciliation.
   - **c.** Pulmonary oedema.
   - **d.** Cranioventral pulmonary consolidation (CVPC).
3. **What is the effect of the inflammatory response to *M. hyopneumoniae*?**
   - **a.** Tissue damage and constriction of the airways.
   - **b.** Rapid and effective elimination of the pathogen.
   - **c.** If a strong humoral (antibody) response develops, there will probably not be any damage to the lungs.
   - **d.** It has no effect on the pathogenesis of the disease.
4. **How is porcine enzootic pneumonia (EP) differentiated from porcine respiratory disease complex (PRDC)?**
   - **a.** *M. hyopneumoniae* is the primary agent for EP, but never for PRDC.
   - **b.** Viral agents are involved in EP.
   - **c.** PRDC tends to be more severe due to the involvement of viral agents.
   - **d.** Porcine respiratory and reproductive syndrome virus (PRRSV) is always involved in PRDC.

5. **Which is the correct answer for *M. hyopneumoniae* infection?**
   a. Lung lesions only develop when there is coinfection with other pig pathogens.
   b. It can occur in pigs of any age.
   c. The individual develops lung lesions whenever infection occurs.
   d. Infection is short-lived and the pathogen is rarely detected 4 weeks after the initial infection.
6. **Complete the sentence: Clinical signs of *M. hyopneumoniae* infection...**
   a. ...are specific to *M. hyopneumoniae*.
   b. ...usually appear in piglets before weaning.
   c. ...are characterised by a dry, persistent and nonproductive cough.
   d. ...are associated with high mortality rates.
7. **What is the approximate incubation time between exposure to *M. hyopneumoniae* and the onset of clinical signs?**
   a. 3–5 days.
   b. 1 week.
   c. 2–6 weeks.
   d. 8–12 weeks.
8. **Which is the correct answer in relation to the forms of porcine enzootic pneumonia (EP)?**
   a. In Europe, the epidemic form is more common than the endemic form.
   b. Both forms are often seen in fattening pigs.
   c. Both forms involve a dry nonproductive cough that affects the whole herd uniformly.
   d. The endemic form is accompanied by a higher mortality rate.

9. Where do the lung lesions associated with *M. hyopneumoniae* infection usually appear?

a. In the apical and cardiac lobes of the lung.

b. In the diaphragmatic lobes of the lung.

c. Only in the accessory lobe of the lung.

d. They affect at least 50 % of the lung surface.

10. Which one of the following images shows lung lesions consistent with *M. hyopneumoniae* infection?

a.

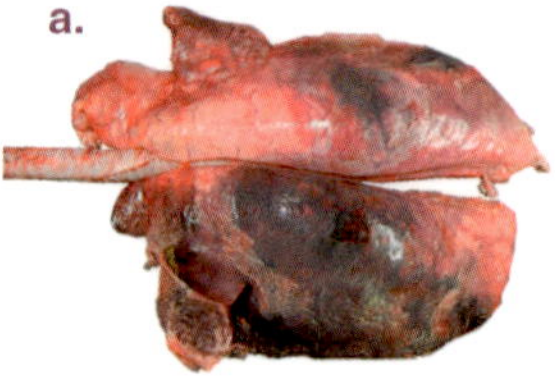

b.

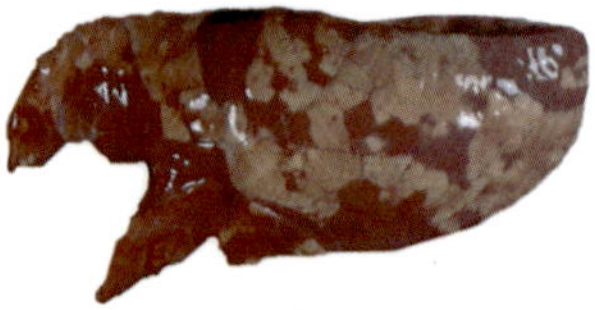

c.

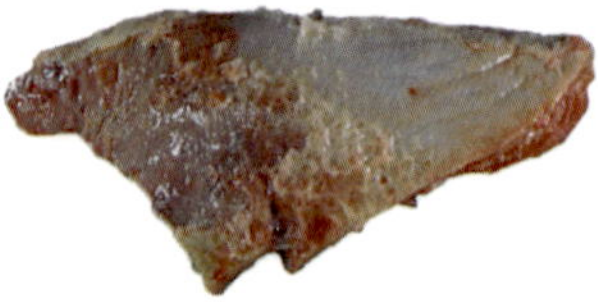

d.

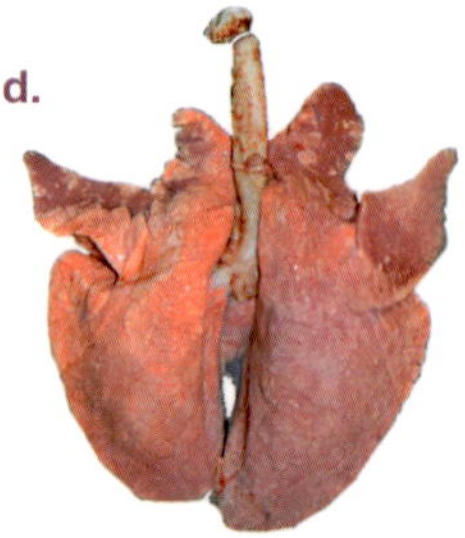

11. Which is the correct answer with respect to the laboratory techniques used to diagnose *M. hyopneumoniae* infection?

a. Immunohistochemistry (IHC), immunofluorescence (IF) and in situ hybridisation (ISH) are performed on lung tissue and allow the presence of *M. hyopneumoniae* to be correlated with the lung lesion.

b. Bacterial culture is the technique of choice for routine diagnosis.

c. A negative result for *M. hyopneumoniae* directly rules out the pathogen.

d. ISH detects the *M. hyopneumoniae* antigen, but IHC and IF detect genetic material (DNA) in the lung tissue.

12. Complete the sentence: In *M. hyopneumoniae* diagnosis, PCR...

a. ...detects antibodies, so it is the best technique to detect seroconversion.
b. ...is only run as it is performed on lung tissue.
c. ...is the best technique to detect the moment of infection.
d. ...is a very specific, but not very sensitive, technique.

13. Which of the following statements is false?

a. Real-time or quantitative PCR enables strains of *M. hyopneumoniae* to be differentiated genetically.
b. One of the most commonly used techniques to detect *M. hyopneumoniae* variability analyses the variable number tandem repeats in certain gene sequences.
c. One individual can be infected by multiple strains of *M. hyopneumoniae*.
d. Up to 13 different strains of *M. hyopneumoniae* have been detected in one batch of pigs.

14. How does *M. hyopneumoniae* variability affect development of the infection?

a. Experimentally, strains of *M. hyopneumoniae* have been classified as having either high or low virulence.
b. In infections by strains of low virulence, the inflammatory response is very strong, so lung lesions are less severe.
c. In infections by strains of high virulence, seroconversion occurs later (further from the moment of infection).
d. Strains of low virulence do not colonise the upper respiratory tract of the pig.

15. Which of these is NOT considered to be a risk factor for *M. hyopneumoniae* infection?

a. Continuous flow production system.
b. Early weaning (under 3 weeks of age).
c. Proximity to other pig farms.
d. Frequent introduction of replacement gilts.

16. Which is the correct answer for gilt acclimatisation?

a. In Europe, exposure to cull sows is the most common acclimatisation procedure.

b. It has no effect on EP development during the fattening stage.

c. It is used to reduce the prevalence of *M. hyopneumoniae* colonisation in piglets.

d. It is not worth doing if litters are weaned early.

17. Which is the correct answer for *M. hyopneumoniae* infection control?

a. Aminoglycosides are the antibiotic of choice.

b. Vaccination reduces clinical signs, lung lesions and minimises the effect on production parameters.

c. Vaccination is sufficient, as it interrupts the transmission of *M. hyopneumoniae* from infected to susceptible animals.

d. The level of serum antibodies resulting from vaccination is directly proportional to the degree of protection against the disease.

18. Which is the correct answer for commercial *M. hyopneumoniae* vaccines?

a. They are all based on *M. hyopneumoniae* strains 11 or J, as these are the reference strains.

b. They are all attenuated live vaccines.

c. They can induce an antibody response even when maternal antibodies are present.

d. They should not be administered for the first time before weaning (3 weeks of age).

19. Which is the correct answer for *M. hyopneumoniae* elimination protocols?

a. The Swiss method is based on the fact that *M. hyopneumoniae* is mostly maintained on the farm by young animals, so animals under 20 months of age are removed from the farm.

b. Complete depopulation, followed by repopulation with individuals that are negative for *M. hyopneumoniae*, is the most successful and commonly used method.

c. The only protocol that does not cause production losses is medication of the whole herd.

d. Mass vaccination of piglets, replacement gilts and breeding sows eliminates *M. hyopneumoniae* infection without the need for antibiotics or other measures.

20. Which is the correct answer for elimination protocols that use herd closure and medication?

a. All animals under 8 months old are removed.

b. Herd closure starts when the first *M. hyopneumoniae* vaccine is administered to the replacement gilts newly admitted.

c. After herd closure, all animals are treated with antibiotics but they are never vaccinated.

d. The 8-month closure is based on data that suggest that this is the minimum period required to ensure that animals have stopped excreting *M. hyopneumoniae* after infection.

SELF-ASSESSMENT

Mark your answers and clarify any doubts.

1. **Answer c: They lack cell walls.** Some antibiotics, such as the β-lactams (penicillin and derivatives) affect cell wall synthesis. Mycoplasmas are resistant to these, as they do not have cell wall.

2. **Answer b: Ciliostasis and deciliation.** Colonization of the pig's respiratory tract is essential to start the infection. *M. hyopneumoniae* penetrates the airways and adheres mainly to the cilia of the epithelial cells, causing ciliostasis (loss of motility) and deciliation (loss of cilia).

3. **Answer a: Tissue damage and constriction of the airways.** One important characteristic of *M. hyopneumoniae* infection is the inflammatory response that is generated. As the infection advances, immune cells are mobilised to the site of the infection. The accumulation of these cells in the airways restricts air flow. This local inflammatory response tends to become chronic, and it is also closely linked to the development of lung lesions.

4. **Answer c: PRDC tends to be more severe due to the involvement of viral agents.** *M. hyopneumoniae* is considered to be a primary pathogen, although its role in porcine respiratory disease is usually related to its interaction with other pathogens. PRDC involves coinfection by multiple pathogens, both viral and bacterial, sometimes including *M. hyopneumoniae*. PRDC tends to be more severe than EP, as it involves viruses as well as the bacteria that are commonly involved in EP.

5. **Answer b: It can occur in pigs of any age.** *M. hyopneumoniae* and its associated diseases are most common in fattening pigs, but pigs of all ages are susceptible to the pathogen.

6. **Answer c: ...are characterised by a dry, persistent and nonproductive cough.** A nonproductive dry cough is suggestive of, but not exclusive to, *M. hyopneumoniae* infection.

7. **Answer c: 2–6 weeks.** Under experimental conditions, coughing tends to start 2 weeks postinfection. However, this period can vary considerably in the field, and can be as long as 6 weeks.

8. **Answer b: Both forms are often seen in fattening pigs.** Regardless of the form (endemic or epidemic), EP usually appears during fattening, but the epidemic form can affect animals of all ages and production stages.

9. **Answer a: In the apical and cardiac lobes of the lung.** Lung lesions associated with *M. hyopneumoniae* consist of consolidation that mainly affects the cranioventral regions of the lung, i.e., the apical and cardiac lobes, and the cranial regions of the diaphragmatic lobes.

10. **Answer d:** This image is a dorsal view of a pig lung showing lesions consistent with *M. hyopneumoniae* infection: bilateral cranioventral pulmonary consolidation (CVPC), affecting the right and left apical and cardiac lobes of the lungs.

d.

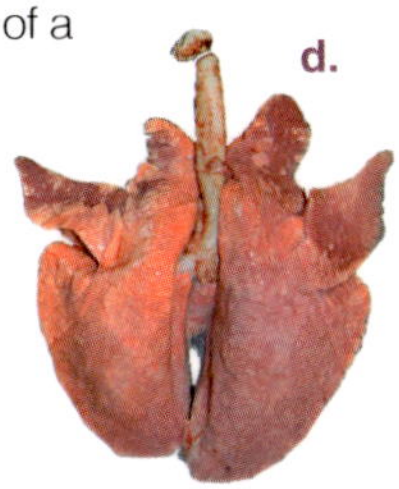

11. **Answer a: Immunohistochemistry (IHC), immunofluorescence (IF) and in situ hybridisation (ISH) are performed on lung tissue and allow the presence of *M. hyopneumoniae* to be correlated with the lung lesion.** IHC and IF detect the *M. hyopneumoniae* antigen (using antibodies), but ISH detects *M. hyopneumoniae* DNA. These techniques are all exclusively used postmortem, as they are run on lung tissue. Their main advantage is that they enable the presence of *M. hyopneumoniae* to be matched to the lung damage seen.

12. **Answer c: …is the best technique to detect the moment of infection.** PCR detects *M. hyopneumoniae* nucleic acids (DNA). It can be used ante and postmortem, as it can be run on a variety of samples. It is also highly sensitive and specific. PCR tests can potentially detect *M. hyopneumoniae* in the first stages of infection, even before a detectable immune response develops and/or there are any clinical signs.

13. **Answer a: Real-time or quantitative PCR enables strains of *M. hyopneumoniae* to be differentiated genetically.** Real-time or quantitative PCR enables DNA to be quantified, but it does not detect *M. hyopneumoniae* variability. Genotyping techniques are required for this.

14. **Answer a: Experimentally, strains of *M. hyopneumoniae* have been classified as having either high or low virulence.** The immune response to *M. hyopneumoniae* has an important effect on lung lesion development. Experimentally, the most virulent strains have been seen to induce stronger local inflammatory immune responses and they usually induce seroconversion sooner. This does not mean that low virulence strains do not colonise the upper respiratory tract and infect the pig.

15. **Answer b: Early weaning (under 3 weeks of age).** The longer the lactation period, the greater the risk of litters being colonised by *M. hyopneumoniae*. Early weaning (under 3 weeks of age) can reduce *M. hyopneumoniae* transmission from the sow to her progeny.

16. **Answer c: It is used to reduce the prevalence of *M. hyopneumoniae* colonisation in piglets.** Good gilt acclimatisation is essential for effective management of *M. hyopneumoniae* on farm. Effective gilt acclimatisation should reduce *M. hyopneumoniae* excretion at first farrowing, resulting in lower piglet colonisation by weaning, which may then lead to fewer respiratory problems during the fattening stage.

17. **Answer b: Vaccination reduces clinical signs, lung lesions and minimises the effect on production parameters.** However, vaccination does not prevent colonisation entirely, and only slightly reduces *M. hyopneumoniae* transmission. EP cannot be controlled by vaccination alone.

18. **Answer c: They can induce an antibody response even when maternal antibodies are present.** Most commercial vaccines are bacterins (inactivated *M. hyopneumoniae* cells) based on different strains of *M. hyopneumoniae* (including reference strains J and 11). There are various vaccination protocols and, in the case of *M. hyopneumoniae*, some studies have demonstrated that commercial vaccines can be effective and induce an antibody response even in the presence of maternal antibodies.

19. **Answer c: The only protocol that does not cause production losses is medication of the whole herd.** The most direct method of eliminating *M. hyopneumoniae* is complete depopulation, followed by repopulation with negative individuals, but one of the most widely used methods used for this pathogen is the Swiss method, where all animals under 10 months old are removed from the farm. Other eradication protocols have been developed to minimise

production losses, including herd closure and medication, or medication alone.

20. **Answer d: The 8-month closure is based on data that suggest that this is the minimum period required to ensure that animals have stopped excreting *M. hyopneumoniae* after infection.** In elimination protocols that employ herd closure and medication, the replacement gilts newly admitted should be exposed to *M. hyopneumoniae,* and once they are confirmed positive for the pathogen, the farm should be closed for approximately 8 months (regardless of when these gilts are vaccinated against *M. hyopneumoniae*). No animals are removed under this protocol, and all animals are medicated and vaccinated once the farm has been closed.

REFERENCES

ANDREASEN, M., MOUSING, J., KROGSGAARD THOMSEN, L., 2001. No simple association between time elapsed from seroconversion until slaughter and the extent of lung lesions in Danish swine. *Prev Vet Med* 52, 147-161.

ARSENAKIS, I., PANZAVOLTA, L., MICHIELS, A., DEL POZO SACRISTÁN, R., BOYEN, F., HAESEBROUCK, F., MAES, D., 2016. Efficacy of *Mycoplasma hyopneumoniae* vaccination before and at weaning against experimental challenge infection in pigs. *BMC Vet Res* 12, 63.

BATISTA, L., PIJOAN, C., RUIZ, A., UTRERA, V., DEE, S., 2004. Assessment of transmission of *Mycoplasma hyopneumoniae* by personnel. *J Swine Health Prod* 12, 75-77.

BLANCHARD, B., VENA, M.M., CAVALIER, A., LE LANNIC, J., GOURANTON, J., KOBISCH, M., 1992. Electron microscopic observation of the respiratory tract of SPF piglets inoculated with *Mycoplasma hyopneumoniae*. *Vet Microbiol* 30, 329-341.

BROWNE, C., LOEFFLER, A., HOLT, H.R., CHANG, Y.M., LLOYD, D.H., NEVEL, A., 2017. Low temperature and dust favour in vitro survival of *Mycoplasma hyopneumoniae*: time to revisit indirect transmission in pig housing. *Lett Appl Microbiol* 64, 2-7.

CALSAMIGLIA, M., COLLINS, J.E., PIJOAN, C., 2000. Correlation between the presence of enzootic pneumonia lesions and detection of *Mycoplasma hyopneumoniae* in bronchial swabs by PCR. *Vet Microbiol* 76, 299-303.

CALSAMIGLIA, M., PIJOAN, C., 2000. Colonisation state and colostral immunity to *Mycoplasma hyopneumoniae* of different parity sows. *Vet Rec* 146, 530-532.

CALUS, D., MAES, D., MEYNS, T., PASMANS, F., HAESEBROUCK, F., 2009. In vivo virulence of *Mycoplasma hyopneumoniae* isolates does not correlate with in vitro adhesion assessed by a microtitre plate adherence assay. *J Appl Microbiol* 106, 1951-1956.

CHARLEBOIS, A., MAROIS-CREHAN, C., HELIE, P., GAGNON, C.A., GOTTSCHALK, M., ARCHAMBAULT, M., 2014. Genetic diversity of *Mycoplasma hyopneumoniae* isolates of abattoir pigs. *Vet Microbiol* 168, 348-356.

DEBEY, M.C., ROSS, R.F., 1994. Ciliostasis and loss of cilia induced by *Mycoplasma hyopneumoniae* in porcine tracheal organ cultures. *Infect Immun* 62, 5312-5318.

DJORDJEVIC, S.P., EAMENS, G.J., ROMALIS, L.F., NICHOLLS, P.J., TAYLOR, V., CHIN, J., 1997. Serum and mucosal antibody responses and protection in pigs vaccinated against *Mycoplasma hyopneumoniae* with vaccines containing a denatured membrane antigen pool and adjuvant. *Aust Vet J* 75, 504-511.

DOS SANTOS, L.F., SREEVATSAN, S., TORREMORELL, M., MOREIRA, M.A., SIBILA, M., PIETERS, M., 2015. Genotype distribution of *Mycoplasma hyopneumoniae* in swine herds from different geographical regions. *Vet Microbiol* 175, 374-381.

FABLET, C., MAROIS-CREHAN, C., SIMON, G., GRASLAND, B., JESTIN, A., KOBISCH, M., MADEC, F., ROSE, N., 2012. Infectious agents associated with respiratory diseases in 125 farrow-to-finish pig herds: a cross-sectional study. *Vet Microbiol* 157, 152-163.

FABLET, C., MAROIS, C., KOBISCH, M., MADEC, F., ROSE, N., 2010. Estimation of the sensitivity of four sampling methods for *Mycoplasma hyopneumoniae* detection in live pigs using a Bayesian approach. *Vet Microbiol* 143, 238-245.

FANO, E., PIJOAN, C., DEE, S., 2005. Dynamics and persistence of *Mycoplasma hyopneumoniae* infection in pigs. *Can J Vet Res* 69, 223-228.

FANO, E., PIJOAN, C., DEE, S., DEEN, J., 2007. Effect of *Mycoplasma hyopneumoniae* colonization at weaning on disease severity in growing pigs. *Can J Vet Res* 71, 195-200.

FRAILE, L., ALEGRE, A., LÓPEZ-JIMÉNEZ, R., NOFRARIAS, M., SEGALÉS, J., 2010. Risk factors associated with pleuritis and cranio-ventral pulmonary consolidation in slaughter-aged pigs. *Vet J* 184, 326-333.

GARCIA-MORANTE, B., SEGALÉS, J., FRAILE, L., PÉREZ DE ROZAS, A., MAITI H., COLL, T., SIBILA, M., 2016. Assessment of *Mycoplasma hyopneumoniae*-induced pneumonia using different lung lesion scoring systems: a comparative review. *J Comp Pathol* 154, 125-34.

GARCIA-MORANTE, B., SEGALÉS, J., SIBILA, M., 2015. La importancia de las cepas de *Mycoplasma hyopneumoniae*. *Suis* nº 115, marzo 2015.

GARZA-MORENO, L., SEGALÉS, J., PIETERS, M., ROMAGOSA, A., SIBILA, M., 2017. Survey on *Mycoplasma hyopneumoniae* gilt acclimation practices in Europe. *Porcine Health Manag* 21, 3-21.

GROSSE BEILAGE, E., ROHDE, N., KRIETER, J., 2009. Seroprevalence and risk factors associated with seropositivity in sows from 67 herds in north-west Germany infected with *Mycoplasma hyopneumoniae*. *Prev Vet Med* 88, 255-263.

Holst, S., Yeske, P., Pieters, M., 2015. Elimination of *Mycoplasma hyopneumoniae* from breed-to-wean farms: A review of current protocols with emphasis on herd closure and medication. *J Swine Health Prod* 23, 321-330.

Kobisch, M., Blanchard, B., Le Potier, M.F., 1993. *Mycoplasma hyopneumoniae* infection in pigs: duration of the disease and resistance to reinfection. *Vet Res* 24, 67-77.

Kobisch, M., Friis, N.F., 1996. Swine mycoplasmoses. *Rev Sci Tech* 15, 1569-1605.

Kurth, K.T., Hsu, T., Snook, E.R., Thacker, E.L., Thacker, B.J., Minion, F.C., 2002. Use of a *Mycoplasma hyopneumoniae* nested polymerase chain reaction test to determine the optimal sampling sites in swine. *J Vet Diagn Invest* 14, 463-469.

Leon, E.A., Madec, F., Taylor, N.M., Kobisch, M., 2001. Seroepidemiology of *Mycoplasma hyopneumoniae* in pigs from farrow-to-finish farms. *Vet Microbiol* 78, 331-341.

Liu, W., Xiao, S., Li, M., Guo, S., Li, S., Luo, R., Feng, Z., Li, B., Zhou, Z., Shao, G., Chen, H., Fang, L., 2013. Comparative genomic analyses of *Mycoplasma hyopneumoniae* pathogenic 168 strain and its high-passaged attenuated strain. *BMC Genomics* 14, 80.

Maes, D., Segalés, J., Meyns, T., Sibila, M., Pieters, M., Haesebrouck, F., 2008. Control of *Mycoplasma hyopneumoniae* infections in pigs. *Vet Microbiol* 126, 297-309.

Maes, D., Sibila, M., Kuhnert, P., Segalés, J., Haesebrouck, F., Pieters, M., 2017. Update on *Mycoplasma hyopneumoniae* infections in pigs: Knowledge gaps for improved disease control. *Transbound Emerg Dis* 23.

Maes, D., Verdonck, M., Deluyker, H., de Kruif, A., 1996. Enzootic pneumonia in pigs. *Vet Q* 18, 104-109.

Mayor, D., Jores, J., Korczak, B.M., Kuhnert, P., 2008. Multilocus sequence typing (MLST) of *Mycoplasma hyopneumoniae:* a diverse pathogen with limited clonality. *Vet Microbiol* 127, 63-72.

Mayor, D., Zeeh, F., Frey, J., Kuhnert, P., 2007. Diversity of *Mycoplasma hyopneumoniae* in pig farms revealed by direct molecular typing of clinical material. *Vet Res* 38, 391-398.

Merialdi, G., Dottori, M., Bonilauri, P., Luppi, A., Gozio, S., Pozzi, P., Spaggiari, B., Martelli, P., 2012. Survey of pleuritis and pulmonary lesions in pigs at abattoir with a focus on the extent of the condition and herd risk factors. *Vet J* 193, 234-239.

Meyns, T., Dewulf, J., de Kruif, A., Calus, D., Haesebrouck, F., Maes, D., 2006. Comparison of transmission of *Mycoplasma hyopneumoniae* in vaccinated and non-vaccinated populations. *Vaccine* 24, 7081-7086.

Meyns, T., Maes, D., Calus, D., Ribbens, S., Dewulf, J., Chiers, K., de Kruif, A., Cox, E., Decostere, A., Haesebrouck, F., 2007. Interactions of highly and low virulent *Mycoplasma hyopneumoniae* isolates with the respiratory tract of pigs. *Vet Microbiol* 120, 87-95.

Meyns, T., Maes, D., Dewulf, J., Vicca, J., Haesebrouck, F., de Kruif, A., 2004. Quantification of the spread of *Mycoplasma hyopneumoniae* in nursery pigs using transmission experiments. *Prev Vet Med* 66, 265-275.

Meyns, T., Van Steelant, J., Rolly, E., Dewulf, J., Haesebrouck, F., Maes, D., 2011. A cross-sectional study of risk factors associated with pulmonary lesions in pigs at slaughter. *Vet J* 187, 388-392.

Michiels, A., Vranckx, K., Piepers, S., Del Pozo Sacristán, R., Arsenakis, I., Boyen, F., Haesebrouck, F., Maes, D., 2017. Impact of diversity of *Mycoplasma hyopneumoniae* strains on lung lesions in slaughter pigs. *Vet Res* 48, 2.

Moorkamp, L., Hewicker-Trautwein, M., Grosse Beilage, E., 2009. Occurrence of *Mycoplasma hyopneumoniae* in coughing piglets (3-6 weeks of age) from 50 herds with a history of endemic respiratory disease. *Transbound Emerg Dis* 56, 54-56.

Morris, C.R., Gardner, I.A., Hietala, S.K., Carpenter, T.E., Anderson, R.J., Parker, K.M., 1995b. Seroepidemiologic study of natural transmission of *Mycoplasma hyopneumoniae* in a swine herd. *Prev Vet Med* 21, 323-337.

Nathues, H., Chang, Y.M., Wieland, B., Rechter, G., Spergser, J., Rosengarten, R., Kreienbrock, L., Grosse Beilage, E., 2014. Herd-level risk factors for the seropositivity to *Mycoplasma hyopneumoniae* and the occurrence of enzootic pneumonia among fattening pigs in areas of endemic infection and high pig density. *Transbound Emerg Dis* 61, 316-328.

Nathues, H., Grosse Beilage, E., Kreienbrock, L., Rosengarten, R., Spergser, J., 2011. RAPD and VNTR analyses demonstrate genotypic heterogeneity of

Mycoplasma hyopneumoniae isolates from pigs housed in a region with high pig density. *Vet Microbiol* 152, 338-345.

Nathues, H., Woeste, H., Doehring, S., Fahrion, A.S., Doherr, M.G., Beilage, E., 2013. Herd specific risk factors for *Mycoplasma hyopneumoniae* infections in suckling pigs at the age of weaning. *Acta Vet Scand* 55, 30.

Noyes, E.P., Feeney, D.A., Pijoan, C., 1990. Comparison of the effect of pneumonia detected during lifetime with pneumonia detected at slaughter on growth in swine. *J Am Vet Med Assoc* 197, 1025-1029.

Opriessnig, T., Gimenez-Lirola, L.G., Halbur, P.G., 2011. Polymicrobial respiratory disease in pigs. *Anim Health Res Rev* 12, 133-148.

Otake, S., Dee, S., Corzo, C., Oliveira, S., Deen, J., 2010. Long-distance airborne transport of infectious PRRSV and *Mycoplasma hyopneumoniae* from a swine population infected with multiple viral variants. *Vet Microbiol* 145, 198-208.

Pantoja, L.G., Pettit, K., Dos Santos, L.F., Tubbs, R., Pieters, M., 2016. *Mycoplasma hyopneumoniae* genetic variability within a swine operation. *J Vet Diagn Invest* 28, 175-179.

Pieters, M., Daniels, J., Rovira, A., 2017. Comparison of sample types and diagnostic methods for in vivo detection of *Mycoplasma hyopneumoniae* during early stages of infection. *Vet Microbiol* 203, 103-109.

Pieters, M., Fano, E., 2016. *Mycoplasma hyopneumoniae* management in gilts. *Vet Rec* 178, 122-123.

Pieters, M., Fano, E., Pijoan, C., Dee, S., 2010. An experimental model to evaluate *Mycoplasma hyopneumoniae* transmission from asymptomatic carriers to unvaccinated and vaccinated sentinel pigs. *Can J Vet Res* 74, 157-160.

Pieters, M., Pijoan, C., Fano, E., Dee, S., 2009. An assessment of the duration of *Mycoplasma hyopneumoniae* infection in an experimentally infected population of pigs. *Vet Microbiol* 134, 261-266.

Pieters, M., Sibila, M., 2017. When is the best time to vaccinate piglets against *Mycoplasma hyopneumoniae*. *Vet Rec* 181, 16-17.

Pinto, P.M., Klein, C.S., Zaha, A., Ferreira, H.B., 2009. Comparative proteomic analysis of pathogenic and non-pathogenic strains from the swine pathogen *Mycoplasma hyopneumoniae*. *Proteome Sci* 7, 45.

Rautiainen, E., Oravainen, J., Virolainen, J.V., Tuovinen, V., 2001. Regional eradication of *Mycoplasma hyopneumoniae* from pig herds and documentation of freedom of the disease. *Acta Vet Scand* 42, 355-364.

Razin, S., Glaser, G., Amikam, D., 1984. Molecular and biological features of mollicutes (mycoplasmas). *Ann Microbiol* (Paris) 135a, 9-15.

Redondo, E., Masot, A.J., Fernández, A., Gázquez, A., 2009. Histopathological and immunohistochemical findings in the lungs of pigs infected experimentally with *Mycoplasma hyopneumoniae*. *J Comp Pathol* 140, 260-270.

Roos, L.R., Fano, E., Homwong, N., Payne, B., Pieters, M., 2016. A model to investigate the optimal seeder-to-naïve ratio for successful natural *Mycoplasma hyopneumoniae* gilt exposure prior to entering the breeding herd. *Vet Microbiol* 184, 51-58.

Rose, D.L., Tully, J.G., Wittler, R.G., 1979. Taxonomy of some swine mycoplasmas: *Mycoplasma suipneumoniae* Goodwin et al. 1965, a later, objective synonym of *Mycoplasma hyopneumoniae* Maré and Switzer 1965, and the status of *Mycoplasma flocculare* Meyling and Friis, 1972. *Int J Syst Evol Microbiol* 29, 83-91.

Sibila, M., Bernal, R., Torrents, D., Riera, P., Llopart, D., Calsamiglia, M., Segalés, J., 2008. Effect of sow vaccination against *Mycoplasma hyopneumoniae* on sow and piglet colonization and seroconversion, and pig lung lesions at slaughter. *Vet Microbiol* 127, 165-170.

Sibila, M., Calsamiglia, M., Segalés, J., Rosell, C., 2004. Association between *Mycoplasma hyopneumoniae* at different respiratory sites and presence of histopathological lung lesions. *Vet Rec* 155, 57-58.

Sibila, M., Nofrarias, M., López-Soria, S., Segalés, J., Riera, P., Llopart, D., Calsamiglia, M., 2007a. Exploratory field study on *Mycoplasma hyopneumoniae* infection in suckling pigs. *Vet Microbiol* 121, 352-356.

Sibila, M., Nofrarias, M., López-Soria, S., Segalés, J., Valero, O., Espinal, A., Calsamiglia, M., 2007b. Chronological study of *Mycoplasma hyopneumoniae* infection, seroconversion and associated lung lesions in vaccinated and non-vaccinated pigs. *Vet Microbiol* 122, 97-107.

Sibila, M., Pieters, M., Molitor, T., Maes, D., Haesebrouck, F., Segalés, J., 2009. Current perspectives on the diagnosis and epidemiology of *Mycoplasma hyopneumoniae* infection. *Vet J* 181, 221-231.

Sitjar, M., Noyes, E.P., Simon, X., Pijoan, C., 1996. Relationship among seroconversion to *Mycoplasma hyopneumoniae*, lung lesions, and production parameters in pigs. *Swine Health Prod* 4, 273-277.

Sørensen, V., Ahrens, P., Barfod, K., Feenstra, A.A., Feld, N.C., Friis, N.F., Bille-Hansen, V., Jensen, N.E., Pedersen, M.W., 1997. *Mycoplasma hyopneumoniae* infection in pigs: duration of the disease and evaluation of four diagnostic assays. *Vet Microbiol* 54, 23-34.

Stakenborg, T., Vicca, J., Butaye, P., Maes, D., Peeters, J., de Kruif, A., Haesebrouck, F., 2005. The diversity of *Mycoplasma hyopneumoniae* within and between herds using pulsed-field gel electrophoresis. *Vet Microbiol* 109, 29-36.

Stärk, K.D., Miserez, R., Siegmann, S., Ochs, H., Infanger, P., Schmidt, J., 2007. A successful national control programme for enzootic respiratory diseases in pigs in Switzerland. *Rev Sci Tech* 26, 595-606.

Thacker, E.L., 2004. Diagnosis of *Mycoplasma hyopneumoniae. Anim Health Res Rev* 5, 317-320.

Thacker, E.L., Minion, F.C., 2012. Mycoplasmosis, In: *Diseases of swine*, 10th ed. Wiley-Blackwell, pp. 779-797.

Thacker, E.L., Thacker, B.J., Boettcher, T.B., Jayappa, H., 1998. Comparison of antibody production, lymphocyte stimulation, and protection induced by four commercial *Mycoplasma hyopneumoniae* bacterins. *J Swine Health Prod* 6, 107-112.

Vicca, J., Stakenborg, T., Maes, D., Butaye, P., Peeters, J., de Kruif, A., Haesebrouck, F., 2003. Evaluation of virulence of *Mycoplasma hyopneumoniae* field isolates. *Vet Microbiol* 97, 177-190.

Villarreal, I., Maes, D., Meyns, T., Gebruers, F., Calus, D., Pasmans, F., Haesebrouck, F., 2009. Infection with a low virulent *Mycoplasma hyopneumoniae* isolate does not protect piglets against subsequent infection with a highly virulent *M. hyopneumoniae* isolate. *Vaccine* 27, 1875-1879.

Villarreal, I., Meyns, T., Dewulf, J., Vranckx, K., Calus, D., Pasmans, F., Haesebrouck, F., Maes, D., 2011. The effect of vaccination on the transmission of *Mycoplasma hyopneumoniae* in pigs under field conditions. *Vet J* 188, 48-52.

Villarreal, I., Vranckx, K., Calus, D., Pasmans, F., Haesebrouck, F., Maes, D., 2012. Effect of challenge of pigs previously immunised with inactivated vaccines containing homologous and heterologous *Mycoplasma hyopneumoniae* strains. *BMC Vet Res* 8, 2.

Vranckx, K., Maes, D., Calus, D., Villarreal, I., Pasmans, F., Haesebrouck, F., 2011. Multiple-locus variable-number tandem-repeat analysis is a suitable tool for differentiation of *Mycoplasma hyopneumoniae* strains without cultivation. *J Clin Microbiol* 49, 2020-2023.

Vranckx, K., Maes, D., Del Pozo Sacristán, R., Pasmans, F., Haesebrouck, F., 2012. A longitudinal study of the diversity and dynamics of *Mycoplasma hyopneumoniae* infections in pig herds. *Vet Microbiol* 156, 315-321.

Wilson, S., Van Brussel, L., Saunders, G., Runnels, P., Taylor, L., Fredrickson, D., Salt, J., 2013. Vaccination of piglets up to 1 week of age with a single-dose *Mycoplasma hyopneumoniae* vaccine induces protective immunity within 2 weeks against virulent challenge in the presence of maternally derived antibodies. *Clin Vaccine Immunol* 20, 720-724.

Wilson, S., Van Brussel, L., Saunders, G., Taylor, L., Zimmermann, L., Heinritzi, K., Ritzmann, M., Banholzer, E., Eddicks, M., 2012. Vaccination of piglets at 1 week of age with an inactivated *Mycoplasma hyopneumoniae* vaccine reduces lung lesions and improves average daily gain in body weight. *Vaccine* 30, 7625-7629.

Woolley, L.K., Fell, S., Gonsalves, J.R., Walker, M.J., Djordjevic, S.P., Jenkins, C., Eamens, G.J., 2012. Evaluation of clinical, histological and immunological changes and qPCR detection of *Mycoplasma hyopneumoniae* in tissues during the early stages of mycoplasmal pneumonia in pigs after experimental challenge with two field isolates. *Vet Microbiol* 161, 186-195.

Zielinski, G.C., Ross, R.F., 1993. Adherence of *Mycoplasma hyopneumoniae* to porcine ciliated respiratory tract cells. *Am J Vet Res* 54, 1262-1269.